The Ultimate Illustrated Guide to Chair Yoga for Seniors Over 60

Elevate Mobility, Flexibility, and Balance to Improve Posture and Alignment | Includes 90+ Video Tutorials!

(Series Vol.-2)

JFD Publications

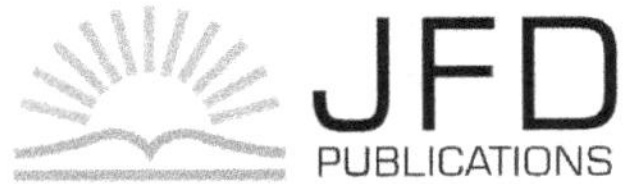

Contents

Introduction

In the quiet moments of reflection, have you ever realized that age is catching up, making once-simple tasks more challenging? You're not alone. Despite the numerous benefits of staying physically active, recent studies reveal a startling truth: approximately 1 in 4 adults aged 50 and older are inactive. (*MMWR Data Highlights* | *Physical Activity* | *CDC,* 2021)

Recent research has shed light on the impact of inactivity, particularly among seniors. For those with obesity, about 31% are often sedentary, and 43% are physically inactive. Such inactivity can lead to various disadvantages, including increased health risks. (Silveira et al., 2022)

As per the Statistica report for 2021, approximately 34.5% of seniors aged 65 or older engaged in no outdoor activities, further emphasizing the importance of addressing sedentary behaviors in this population. (Share of Physically Inactive Population by Age US 2021, n.d.)

On a positive note, another study found that older adults (60 and above) who stay physically active enjoy several benefits. They have a lower risk of heart issues, cancer, fractures, falls, and limitations in daily activities. Being active also helps with better thinking, less chance of memory problems, and a lower risk of feeling down. So, getting into activities like chair yoga can make your life healthier and more fulfilling as you age. (Cunningham et al., 2020)

We Understand Your Struggles

Maintaining an active lifestyle becomes crucial with advancing age, yet we know it can be challenging. Mobility limitations, routine challenges, safety concerns, and the link between mental and physical health can create barriers. We are here to help those facing these challenges and seeking a way to reclaim vitality. We get it, and that's why we have created "The Ultimate Illustrated Guide to Chair Yoga for Seniors Over 60," addressing your unique concerns for a healthier and more vibrant life.

Whether it's struggling to reach a high shelf or finding a favorite activity that is more physically demanding, no matter your catalyst for change, this book will help you. The beauty of chair yoga lies in its versatility; it becomes your solution. You're not alone in this journey, and the path to a more active and fulfilling life begins now with chair yoga as your guiding companion.

Your Shortcut to Success

In this book, we've crafted an empowering 8-step guide to chair yoga, ensuring a seamless path to success:

Understanding Chair Yoga: Explore the history of chair yoga, dispel myths, and grasp safety practices for a confident start.

Setting Up Your Space: Create a dedicated haven for your chair yoga practice, tailored to your preferences.

Fundamental Poses: Master foundational poses, setting the stage for your transformative journey.

Beginner Poses Mastery: Dive into 25 beginner poses, each with detailed guidance to enhance your practice.

Intermediate Poses Mastery: Progress with 25 intermediate poses, achieving a well-rounded and balanced routine.

Advanced Poses Mastery: Challenge yourself with 18 advanced poses guided by expert instructions to elevate your practice.

The 28-Day Challenge: Start a unique 28-day challenge designed to jumpstart your chair yoga journey, fostering consistency and growth.

Beyond the Chair: Explore how chair yoga seamlessly integrates into every facet of your life, making it a continuous and enriching lifestyle.

Each chapter unlocks a new dimension, ensuring your chair yoga experience is tailored, progressive, and, most importantly, enjoyable.

Real Stories, Real Results

Don't just take our word for it. Immerse yourself in the authentic experiences of those who've embraced chair yoga, including renowned celebrities who stand as living testimonials to its transformative power. Here are a few examples from the list of celebrities in their senior years who do yoga and chair yoga to stay fit.

Consider Jane Fonda, the 86-year-old actress and fitness icon. Dealing with chronic pain, arthritis, and osteoporosis, she attributes her resilience to chair yoga, attesting to its impact on both body and mind. (Yoga Stretching & Mobility Workout: PM- Jane Fonda, n.d.)

And let's remember King Charles, the successor to Queen Elizabeth II. At 75, he recognizes the importance of maintaining an active lifestyle, particularly through practices like chair yoga. As he gracefully ages, these exercises support his flexibility, posture, and overall well-being. This highlights the relevance of chair yoga for seniors, demonstrating that individuals from every walk of life find value in its accessible and effective approach. (Charles: The King Who Believes in the Healing Power of Yoga, Ayurveda, n.d.)

These aren't just celebrity endorsements; they are real-life testimonials from individuals, including iconic figures, who've added chair yoga into their daily routines. Their stories echo the transformative power awaiting you in the world of chair yoga.

What Awaits You

Picture a life where age doesn't define your vitality but enhances it. As you enter the chair yoga world through this book, visualize days filled with energy and joy. Feel the ease as you move through life, experiencing newfound flexibility and strength.

Imagine a physically agile future and a mentally resilient one, too. Chair yoga becomes your daily sanctuary—a practice revitalizing body and mind. This healthy future awaits you, a life where age is just a number, and each day brings a renewed sense of well-being.

Why Trust Us

We're not just another publisher but your go-to authority for senior well-being. JFD Publications specializes in crafting top-notch resources exclusively tailored to support the health and happiness of seniors. We know the challenges aging can bring, and we're here to provide the knowledge and tools you need to navigate this journey confidently.

Our commitment to creating engaging and informative materials stems from a genuine understanding of the hurdles that come with aging. We're motivated to empower seniors and caregivers, ensuring they have the resources for a fulfilling and healthy life.

Start Your Chair Yoga Journey

Ready to transform your life through the power of chair yoga? Dive into the comprehensive guide in these pages and begin your journey toward increased mobility, improved flexibility, and enhanced overall well-being. Your vibrant future awaits—seize it with every page you turn. Let's make chair yoga an exercise routine and a lifestyle that elevates your daily experience. Start now and embrace the positive change that chair yoga can bring to your life.

Step #1: Understanding Chair Yoga

"I do as I feel, and I like to stay active and be around people. I still want to keep moving. If I sat down, I think I'd just give up." – Toni Stahl, who works out regularly at age 100!

T*oni's Inspiration:* Toni Stahl's commitment to staying active at the age of 100 is nothing short of inspirational. Her words resonate with the spirit of those who refuse to let age dictate their vitality. Now, let's start the journey that can bring the same energy and enthusiasm into your life through the gentle practice of chair yoga. So, what exactly is chair yoga, and why might it be the perfect fit for you?

What is Chair Yoga?

Chair yoga is a modified form of traditional yoga that incorporates the support of a chair. It brings the benefits of yoga to individuals who may have mobility issues or find it challenging to practice on the floor. The beauty of chair yoga lies in its adaptability, making it accessible to diverse fitness levels.

One of the best things about chair yoga is its simplicity. You only need a sturdy chair with no arms, comfortable clothing, and a space to move around. No fancy equipment or expensive gear is required – just you, a chair, and a willingness to explore.

Why Chair Yoga?

Chair yoga is not just a form of exercise; it's a holistic approach to well-being, perfectly tailored for those in their golden years. It's about promoting mobility, flexibility, and balance safely and enjoyably. This isn't an intense workout that leaves you breathless; it's a gentle, effective practice designed to meet you where you are and guide you toward a healthier and more active lifestyle.

So, if you've ever felt that traditional exercises are too strenuous or intimidating, chair yoga offers a welcoming alternative. It's time to embrace a new way of staying active that aligns with your needs and respects your unique journey. In the following sections, we'll delve deeper into the world of chair yoga, exploring its origin and history, how it differs from traditional yoga, its benefits, and safety tips and precautions when doing it.

How Chair Yoga Differs from Traditional Yoga

In the world of yoga, the beauty lies in its diversity, offering practices that cater to a wide range of individuals. Chair yoga, while rooted in the principles of traditional yoga, presents a unique approach that makes it particularly accessible for seniors. Here is how chair yoga differs from conventional, on-the-mat yoga.

1. **Seated Support:** The most apparent distinction is using a chair. In traditional yoga, practitioners often move through a sequence of poses on a mat, using the floor for support. Chair yoga, on the other hand, integrates the chair as a prop, providing stability and assistance. This seated support makes it feasible for individuals with limited mobility or those uncomfortable with floor exercises to experience the benefits of yoga.

2. **Adapted Poses:** Chair yoga modifies traditional yoga poses to accommodate the seated position. Poses are adjusted to be gentle on joints, making them more accessible for seniors. Traditional yoga may involve complex poses that require getting down on the floor and transitioning between standing and sitting. Chair yoga simplifies these poses, ensuring comfort and safety.

3. **Gentle Movement:** While traditional yoga often involves flowing sequences and dynamic movements, chair yoga focuses on gentle and controlled motions. The emphasis is on enhancing flexibility, improving balance, and promoting relaxation. The pace is tailored to accommodate the comfort level of seniors, allowing for a more enjoyable and accessible experience.

4. **Accessibility:** Traditional yoga classes can sometimes be physically demanding, potentially excluding individuals with certain health conditions or physical limitations. Chair yoga, emphasizing adaptability and accessibility, provides a welcoming environment for all fitness levels. It invites everyone to participate, regardless of their age or physical condition.

5. **Safety and Confidence:** Chair yoga prioritizes safety, addressing concerns that may arise from worries about balance or injury. The chair serves as a stable base, instilling confidence in practitioners. This focus on safety makes chair yoga an ideal choice for those who may have reservations about engaging in traditional yoga practices.

In essence, chair yoga is not a replacement for traditional yoga but a complementary and inclusive alternative. It bridges the gap, ensuring that the enriching benefits of yoga are accessible to seniors who might otherwise feel excluded.

History and Origins of Chair Yoga

Chair yoga may seem like a recent innovation, but its roots trace back to a visionary who recognized the need for inclusivity in the yoga world. Let's uncover chair yoga's fascinating history and origins, exploring when it was created, who pioneered it, and how this gentle practice began.

When it was Created:

The inception of chair yoga can be attributed to the late 20th century, when the traditional image of a yogi was evolving, and the importance of adapting practices to individual needs became increasingly apparent. In the 1980s and 1990s, chair yoga emerged as a response to the growing demand for accessible and modified yoga practices.

By Whom it was Created:

The credit for creating chair yoga goes to Lakshmi Voelker-Binder, a yoga instructor and enthusiast who saw the potential to make yoga more inclusive. Lakshmi, a certified Kripalu Yoga teacher, developed the method of chair yoga in the early 1980s. Her intention was clear: to bring the transformative benefits of yoga to individuals who faced challenges with traditional practices due to age, physical limitations, or health conditions.

How it Began:

Lakshmi's journey into chair yoga started with a deep understanding of the diverse needs within her yoga classes. Witnessing the desire of individuals with mobility issues to experience the joys of yoga, she began adapting traditional poses to be performed while seated. By incorporating a chair as a prop, she not only made yoga accessible but also created a nurturing environment for those who might otherwise feel excluded from the practice.

As chair yoga gained recognition, its appeal expanded beyond seniors and individuals with mobility issues. Its adaptability and gentle approach drew practitioners from various walks of life, establishing chair yoga as a valuable addition to the yogic landscape.

The genesis of chair yoga exemplifies the evolution of yoga as a practice that embraces diversity and strives to meet the unique needs of each individual. Lakshmi Voelker-Binder's pioneering spirit has left an indelible mark on the world of yoga, opening doors for countless individuals to experience this enriching practice's physical, mental, and emotional benefits.

Benefits of Chair Yoga for Seniors

Exercising in your mature years brings lasting benefits, but high-intensity workouts can pose risks as the body ages. The potential for pain and injury increases with longer recovery times. Chair yoga provides a simplified and gentle approach, making it easy for seniors of all fitness levels to engage. Its essence lies in accessibility, allowing individuals with limited mobility or balance concerns to participate comfortably, fostering inclusivity and support in the yoga experience. Other benefits of chair yoga include:

Increased Flexibility

Chair yoga serves as a gentle yet effective method for enhancing flexibility. By incorporating poses that involve stretching the body in unique ways, individuals experience increased flexibility, reaching areas that might need to be addressed regularly. This improves overall mobility, making daily tasks more manageable and promoting a better range of motion.

Improves Muscle Strength

Engaging in chair yoga promotes flexibility and builds and strengthens muscles. The varied poses and movements serve as a low-impact means of toning muscles and enhancing overall strength. This increase in muscle strength supports balance and mobility and serves as a protective measure against potential injuries. A small-scale study involving 35 older women in community care discovered that 12 weeks of chair yoga led to significant improvements in strength, particularly in the hands, arms, and legs. (Yao & Tseng, 2019)

Helps with Balance and Coordination

Chair yoga's focus on spatial awareness during pose transitions improves balance and coordination. The practice encourages mindfulness of different body parts and movements, fostering a deeper connection to one's body. This heightened awareness contributes to enhanced balance and coordination, crucial elements for daily activities.

Reduces Stress

Through intentional breathing and mindful movements, chair yoga provides a valuable avenue for stress reduction. The practice becomes a form of moving meditation, diverting attention from life's stressors. Incorporating moments of meditation during chair yoga further aids in relaxation, offering a respite from the demands of everyday life.

Reduces Pain and Better Pain Management Skills

Regular chair yoga practice releases endorphins, the body's natural painkillers. This not only uplifts mood but also helps alleviate discomfort and pain. A compelling study conducted in 2016 with older adults suffering from osteoarthritis (OA) revealed that an 8-week chair yoga program led to a significant reduction in joint pain. Astonishingly, this positive effect persisted for at least three months after the program concluded, highlighting the enduring benefits of chair yoga in managing and alleviating pain. The focused breathing and controlled movements in chair yoga improve pain management skills, empowering individuals to cope effectively with any discomfort they may experience. (Park et al., 2016)

Promotes Better Sleep

Like other forms of exercise, chair yoga plays a role in regulating the body's sleep-wake cycle. Regular engagement in chair yoga can contribute to better sleep quality. The moderate energy exertion during chair yoga sessions strikes a balance that supports a healthy sleep pattern without inducing fatigue.

Boosts Confidence and Alleviates Depression and Anxiety

Research indicates that chair yoga can have positive effects on mental well-being, including alleviating symptoms of depression and anxiety. The focused and meditative aspects of chair yoga provide a sanctuary for individuals to release negative emotions, fostering a sense of lightness and renewal. As confidence grows through the practice, the overall mood is uplifted.

As we explore the benefits of chair yoga, remember that these advantages extend beyond the physical. Chair yoga addresses the holistic well-being of seniors, promoting a lifestyle that is not only health-conscious but also joyous and fulfilling.

The Broader Applicability of Chair Yoga

Chair yoga transcends its niche, offering benefits that extend far beyond the mat. Let's explore how chair yoga is a versatile and inclusive practice with broader implications for individuals of all ages and abilities.

How Chair Yoga Improves Health Conditions:

Chair yoga is a therapeutic ally, especially for those managing health conditions. The modified poses and gentle movements of chair yoga, which you will learn in this book, cater to individuals with arthritis, osteoporosis, chronic pain, and various physical challenges. Through targeted practices, chair yoga contributes to the alleviation of discomfort, promotes joint flexibility, and enhances overall physical well-being. Scientific studies, including a 2023 research project with older adults suffering from knee osteoarthritis, have highlighted the effectiveness of chair yoga in reducing joint pain, a testament to its positive impact on health conditions. (Yao et al., 2023)

The Impact of Chair Yoga on Mental Health:

The mind-body connection is a cornerstone of chair yoga, offering profound benefits for mental health. Through mindful breathing, meditation, and purposeful movements, chair yoga provides a sanctuary for stress reduction and relaxation. As individuals engage in this practice, they cultivate a sense of calm, fostering mental resilience and a positive outlook.

Chair Yoga is for All Ages:

Age limitations do not confine chair yoga; it is a practice for everyone. Whether you're in your 50s, proactively preparing for the future, or a senior seeking to maintain vitality, chair yoga welcomes participants of all ages. Its adaptability ensures that individuals can tailor the practice to their unique needs and abilities, promoting mobility, balance, and overall physical function.

Chair Yoga is Accessible:

Inclusivity is at the core of chair yoga's appeal. Incorporating a chair as a prop makes the practice accessible to diverse individuals. Whether you have limited mobility, balance concerns, or specific health conditions, chair yoga provides a supportive environment. This accessibility extends beyond physical considerations, embracing individuals at various fitness levels and backgrounds, creating an environment where everyone can experience the enriching benefits of yoga.

Safety Tips and Precautions

Engaging in chair yoga is about reaping the benefits and ensuring a safe and comfortable practice. Here are some safety tips to remember when starting your chair yoga journey.

Avoid Inversions:

Inversion poses, where the head is below the heart, might not suit everyone, especially those with certain health conditions like high blood pressure or glaucoma. It's advisable to skip poses that involve full inversions to prioritize safety and avoid potential complications.

Proper Equipment:

Ensuring the right equipment is crucial for a safe chair yoga practice. Choose a sturdy chair without arms and place it on a non-slip surface to prevent accidents. Additionally, having a yoga block or cushion nearby can provide extra support and comfort during certain poses.

Proper Clothes:

Wearing comfortable and breathable clothing allows for a more enjoyable practice. Loose, stretchy fabrics are ideal, ensuring freedom of movement without restriction. Proper footwear is essential for stability; however, since chair yoga is primarily seated, bare feet or non-slip socks may be preferable for certain individuals.

Listen to Your Body:

One of the most important safety tips is to listen to your body. If a pose causes discomfort or pain, modifying or skipping it is crucial. Chair yoga is about personalizing the practice to suit your needs, so honor your body's signals and adjust accordingly.

Consult with a Healthcare Professional:

Before incorporating any new exercise routine into your lifestyle, mainly if you have existing health conditions, seeking guidance from your healthcare professional is essential. They can offer advice tailored to your health status and confirm whether chair yoga is a secure and appropriate complement to your wellness regimen.

Gradual Progression:

For beginners or those returning to physical activity, gradual progression is critical. Start with basic poses, gradually increasing intensity and complexity as your strength and flexibility improve. This approach minimizes the risk of injury and allows your body to adapt to the practice. We got you covered with 25 exercises for beginners, 25 for intermediate, and 25 for advanced coming up in the following chapters.

Stay Hydrated:

Even though chair yoga is a low-impact practice, staying hydrated is essential. Proper hydration supports overall health and can help prevent issues like muscle cramps. Have water within reach and take sips as needed throughout your session.

Incorporating these safety tips into your chair yoga practice creates a foundation for a secure and enjoyable journey. Remember, the key is to prioritize your well-being, honor your body's needs, and embrace the practice to nurture your physical and mental health.

Addressing Common Concerns and Misconceptions

Embarking on a chair yoga journey may come with specific concerns or misconceptions. Let's address ten common worries and set the record straight, ensuring you approach chair yoga with confidence and enthusiasm.

"I'm Not Flexible Enough for Yoga."

Dispelling the Misconception: Chair yoga is designed to meet you where you are. It's not about extreme flexibility but rather about gentle movements that enhance your current range of motion. The practice adapts to your abilities, promoting flexibility at your own pace.

"Yoga is Only for the Young and Fit."

Dispelling the Misconception: Chair yoga is inclusive and suitable for all ages and fitness levels. It's specially tailored for seniors, offering a gentle yet effective way to stay active. The practice is about well-being, not about fitting into a particular mold.

"I Can't Do Yoga with My Health Condition."

Dispelling the Misconception: Chair yoga is incredibly adaptable. Many health conditions can be accommodated through modified poses. Always consult your healthcare professional; with their guidance, chair yoga can be a safe and beneficial addition to your wellness routine.

"Yoga is Too Intense for Seniors."

Dispelling Misconception: Chair yoga is designed for seniors, considering their unique needs. The practice is gentle, emphasizing gradual progression. It's not about intensity but about promoting mobility, flexibility, and balance at a comfortable pace.

"I Need Expensive Equipment."

Dispelling the Misconception: All you need for chair yoga is a sturdy chair without arms and a clear space to move. No expensive equipment is required. The simplicity of chair yoga is one of its strengths, making it accessible to everyone.

"Yoga Poses are Complicated and Difficult to Remember."

Dispelling the Misconception: Chair yoga poses are intentionally straightforward to remember. The practice emphasizes simplicity and repetition, making it accessible even for those who struggle to remember intricate sequences. We also provided you with the links to videos demonstrating the poses described in this book so you understand the moves and as a reminder if you forget how to do a specific movement.

"I Don't Have Enough Time for Yoga."

Dispelling the Misconception: Chair yoga can be done in short sessions; even 10 min a day can yield benefits. For example, the 28-day challenge in this guide offers a structured yet time-efficient way to incorporate chair yoga into your routine. You will also be able to modify the challenge and do it the following month because, as we saw, after 8 weeks the benefits are lasting.

"Yoga Won't Help with Weight Loss."

Dispelling the Misconception: While chair yoga may not be as calorie-burning as vigorous exercises, it contributes to overall well-being. The practice fosters a mindful and balanced approach to health, which can support weight management as part of a holistic lifestyle. The loss of weight becomes a byproduct of cultivating the habit.

"I'll Feel Awkward or Uncomfortable."

Dispelling the Misconception: Chair yoga is designed to be comfortable and enjoyable. The supportive nature of the chair ensures stability, reducing the risk of discomfort. The practice is about embracing your unique journey, free from judgment.

"Yoga is Only for Spiritual or Religious People."

Dispelling the Misconception: Chair yoga is a versatile practice tailored to individuals with various beliefs. It focuses on yoga's physical and mental benefits without adhering to a specific spiritual or religious philosophy.

As we dispel these common concerns and misconceptions, it's important to approach chair yoga with an open mind and a sense of curiosity. The practice is about your well-being and personal growth. Let go of worries, embrace the journey, and discover the transformative potential of chair yoga in enhancing your life.

. . .

Final Words

As we journey through the understanding of chair yoga, let's reconnect with the inspiring words of Toni Stahl, who, at age 100, champions an active and vibrant lifestyle. Her commitment to staying active reflects the essence of chair yoga— a practice that embraces movement, regardless of age or physical condition.

Key Takeaways

Inclusivity: Chair yoga is an inclusive practice that caters to all ages and fitness levels, encouraging a gentle and adaptable approach to well-being.

Accessible Wisdom: The practice isn't about extremes or unattainable poses. It's a journey toward better health through simple yet impactful movements, emphasizing comfort and individualized progress.

The next chapter will address the practical aspects of starting your chair yoga practice. From creating an inviting space to exploring fundamental poses, chapter two will guide you in establishing the foundation for a fulfilling and transformative chair yoga journey. Get ready to carve out your own space for well-being, where the benefits of chair yoga come to life. Let's continue this exploration with enthusiasm and a commitment to the joyous potential that chair yoga holds for us all.

Step #2: Setting Up Space

"Exercise not only changes your body, it changes your mind, your attitude, and your mood." — Unknown.

Setting up your space in chair yoga is more than arranging furniture; it's crafting a personal retreat where your practice unfolds. Visualize it as a sanctuary that accommodates your body and nurtures positive change. This chapter explores the details of space creation, emphasizing its impact on your physical, mental, and emotional well-being.

Creating your chair yoga space is about cultivating an environment that echoes your intentions. It becomes a stage for your practice, where each pose and breath is an intentional step toward well-being. It is a place where the benefits of chair yoga are not just observed but embraced—a tranquil zone that supports you in every stretch, every pose, and every moment of chair yoga practice. Your space becomes a silent companion through intentional design, inviting positive change.

Creating a Safe and Comfortable Environment

Setting the stage for your chair yoga practice involves some effort. It's about curating a safe and comfortable environment supporting your journey toward well-being. Let's explore detailed guidelines to ensure your space is conducive to a fulfilling chair yoga experience. Note: Of course, you can do this practice outside in a tranquil zone if you have the nice weather for it, just like in the video tutorials we give you access to (with the QR code links in the following chapters)...

Ample Space for Movement

Begin by carving out a space to extend your arms and legs without hindrance freely. Consider chair yoga's full range of motion; this may involve reaching out or stretching your legs. A clear, uncluttered area ensures you can move confidently without worrying about knocking into objects or tripping over items. Take a moment to assess the surroundings and remove any potential stumbling blocks. A spacious zone sets the foundation for an unrestricted, secure chair yoga experience.

For added safety, make sure the surface under your chair is stable and slip-resistant. If you're practicing on a yoga mat, ensure it's firmly in place to prevent any unintended slipping or sliding during your session.

Stable Chair Placement

The stability of your chair is paramount to a safe and effective chair yoga practice. Choose a surface, whether a yoga mat or a non-slip rug, that provides a secure foundation for your chair. Check that the chair's legs are firmly planted and won't shift unexpectedly. Positioning the backrest against a wall adds an extra layer of stability, minimizing the risk of the chair tipping backward during certain poses. Prioritize a stable chair placement to create an environment where you can focus on your practice without any concerns about unexpected movements.

Proper Seating Alignment

How you sit on the chair plays a crucial role in maintaining a safe and aligned practice. Position your chair with its backrest against a wall for added support, ensuring it won't inadvertently move during your movements. As you sit on the chair, pay attention to your posture—maintain a straight spine with your feet planted firmly on the ground. Proper alignment minimizes the risk of strain on your back and joints, allowing you to fully engage in the practice without compromising your safety.

Optimal Lighting

The proper lighting sets the tone for a comfortable and safe chair yoga environment—practice in an area with abundant natural light. Natural light not only enhances visibility but also contributes to an uplifting atmosphere. Opt for soft, ambient lighting that bathes the space in a gentle glow if natural light is scarce. Adequate lighting ensures you can see your surroundings, preventing missteps and creating a welcoming atmosphere for your practice.

Table or Stand for Devices

Many of us turn to digital devices for guided chair yoga sessions in our modern age. If you're following along with instructional videos or virtual classes, having a designated table or stand for your laptop or phone is a more practical approach. Position the device within your line of sight, ensuring you can easily follow instructions without straining your neck. The convenience of having a stable surface for your devices enhances the accessibility of your chair yoga practice, making it seamless and enjoyable.

Comfortable Attire and Flooring

Your clothing and the flooring you practice on contribute significantly to the overall comfort of your chair yoga session. Opt for attire that allows for easy movement, avoiding anything restrictive. If you're practicing on a hard surface, such as hardwood or tile, consider placing a yoga mat or a rug beneath your chair. This provides extra cushioning for your joints, making it more comfortable. The proper attire and flooring choices enable you to fully immerse yourself in the chair yoga experience without any unnecessary discomfort, allowing you to focus on the transformative benefits of the practice.

Background Music or Sounds

Enhance the ambiance of your chair yoga space by adding background music or soothing sounds. Select gentle tunes or nature sounds that complement the meditative aspects of chair yoga. Music can create a calming atmosphere, promote relaxation, and aid focus during practice. Experiment with different genres or sounds to find what resonates with you and enhances the overall experience of your chair yoga session.

Personal Touches

Infuse your chair yoga space with personal touches that uplift and inspire. Whether it's a favorite plant, a small inspirational quote, or calming colors, these elements can contribute to the positive atmosphere of your practice area. Your chair yoga space reflects your unique journey, so make it a place that resonates with positivity and well-being. Consider it your sanctuary, where each pose and breath aligns with the elements that bring you joy and comfort.

By meticulously implementing these guidelines, you're not just creating a space for chair yoga; you're shaping an environment that fosters safety, comfort, and an immersive sense of well-being. Let your chair yoga space be a haven where you can fully embrace the transformative benefits of the practice, promoting positive change and holistic wellness.

Choosing the Right Chair

Selecting the appropriate chair for your practice is fundamental to ensuring a safe and comfortable experience. Let's delve into the key characteristics that make the right chair and explore how to modify an existing one to suit your chair yoga needs better. Additionally, we will highlight chairs to avoid, as certain types may compromise the stability and effectiveness of your practice.

Ideal Chair Characteristics

Sturdy and Stable: Opt for a chair with a solid and stable frame. It should be robust enough to support your weight and provide a secure base for various poses. The absence of wheels or swiveling mechanisms ensures stability and safety during dynamic movements.

Straight Back: Choose a chair with a straight back that offers adequate support to your spine. The backrest should promote a comfortable seated position without encouraging excessive leaning. This ensures proper spinal alignment during your chair yoga practice.

Comfortable Seat: Prioritize a chair with a comfortable, flat seat. This feature allows you to sit evenly without discomfort or imbalance. If the chair has cushions, ensure they complement your movements rather than hinder them.

Armrests: While optional, chairs with sturdy armrests can benefit specific poses.

Ensure that the armrests neither restrict your range of motion nor cause discomfort during practice. They should provide additional support without impeding movement.

Appropriate Height: The chair's height should permit your feet to rest flat on the ground, establishing a stable foundation. Chairs too high or too low can impact your posture and alignment, so selecting the appropriate height is crucial.

Modifying an Existing Chair

If you already have a chair that partially meets the ideal characteristics, consider making modifications to enhance its suitability for chair yoga.

Adding Stability: If your chair lacks stability, place it on a non-slip mat or surface to prevent unnecessary movement. Alternatively, securing the chair against a wall can provide additional support, ensuring a stable foundation for your practice.

Seat Cushion Adjustments: Experiment with adding or removing cushions to adjust the seat's firmness. A balance between comfort and support is recommended for creating an optimal surface for your chair yoga practice.

Back Support: For chairs with insufficient back support, consider using a small cushion or a rolled-up towel to provide additional lumbar support. This modification enhances comfort and helps maintain proper spinal alignment.

Chairs to Avoid

Rolling or Swivel Chairs: Chairs with wheels or swivel are unsuitable for chair yoga. Their lack of stability poses safety risks and may lead to accidents or discomfort during dynamic poses.

Unstable or Flimsy Chairs: Chairs that wobble or feel flimsy should be avoided. Ensuring the chair's structural integrity is vital for your safety and the effectiveness of your chair yoga practice.

Overly Cushioned Chairs: Chairs with excessive cushioning may impede movement and make it challenging to maintain proper alignment. Opt for chairs that balance comfort and support to facilitate a seamless chair yoga experience.

Understanding the key characteristics of the right chair for chair yoga and making necessary modifications ensure a conducive environment for your practice. Avoiding chairs with certain features, such as wheels or instability, fosters a safe and effective chair yoga experience. Remember, your chair is not just a seat; it's a supportive companion on your journey to holistic well-being.

Incorporating Props for Added Support

Enhance your chair yoga practice by incorporating props that provide additional support and deepen the benefits of each pose. Whether you're looking for commercially available props or DIY alternatives, here's a comprehensive list to elevate your chair yoga experience.

Cushions and Pillows

• *Commercial Option:* Yoga-specific cushions or meditation pillows to support your seated poses

• *DIY Alternative:* Utilize firm bed pillows or cushions from your couch to create a comfortable and supportive base for seated postures.

Yoga Blocks

• *Commercial Option:* Standard yoga blocks provide height and stability for various poses

• *DIY Alternative:* Substitute with sturdy books or small, equally-sized boxes to achieve a similar effect.

Resistance Bands

• *Commercial Option:* Light to medium resistance bands can add gentle resistance to your arm and leg exercises.

• *DIY Alternative:* Explore household items like old stretchable garments for improvised resistance

Blankets

• *Commercial Option:* Yoga blankets with a comfortable yet supportive texture

• *DIY Alternative:* Use thick blankets or folded towels to create a soft, supportive surface for seated or reclined poses

Yoga Straps

• *Commercial Option:* Yoga straps assist in achieving proper alignment and stretching during seated and standing poses

• *DIY Alternative:* Substitute with a sturdy belt or long scarf to support stretches and enhance flexibility

Therapy Balls

• *Commercial Option:* Therapy balls for targeted muscle release

• *DIY Alternative:* Utilize tennis balls for self-myofascial release by gently rolling them over tight or sore areas.

Chair Yoga Belt

• *Commercial Option:* Specifically designed belts with buckle closures for seated poses and stretches

• *DIY Alternative:* Craft your belt using a durable fabric or repurpose a belt from your wardrobe

Hand Weights

• *Commercial Option:* Light hand weights for gentle strength training exercises

• *DIY Alternative:* Use water bottles or canned goods as makeshift weights for added resistance

Hand Towels

• *Commercial Option:* Microfiber yoga towels designed for sweat absorption and comfort

• *DIY Alternative:* Regular hand towels can serve the same purpose, providing comfort and moisture control during your practice.

Non-Skid Mat or Rug

• *Commercial Option:* Non-skid yoga mats or rugs to place beneath your chair for added stability

• *DIY Alternative:* Secure a non-slip mat to prevent chair movement on smooth surfaces.

Experiment with these props to discover which ones enhance your chair yoga practice. Whether you choose commercial options or get creative with DIY alternatives, incorporating props can transform your sessions, offering added support and comfort for a more fulfilling experience.

Importance of Proper Posture in Chair Yoga

Maintaining proper posture (aka "correct posture") is a cornerstone of any yoga practice, and chair yoga is no exception. The alignment of your body plays a crucial role in optimizing the benefits of each pose, ensuring safety, and promoting overall health. Here is why proper posture is of utmost importance in chair yoga.

Alignment and Balance

Proper posture in chair yoga is synonymous with correct alignment. Each pose is designed to engage specific muscle groups and promote balance within the body. When you maintain proper posture, you align your spine, hips, and limbs, creating a harmonious balance that fosters stability. This alignment enhances the effectiveness of individual poses and results in an overall sense of equilibrium (aka "balance") during your practice.

Preventing Strain and Discomfort

Chair yoga aims to provide a gentle and accessible exercise, making it suitable for individuals of all fitness levels. Correct posture is instrumental in preventing unnecessary strain on muscles and joints. A study published in the Healthcare Journal emphasizes the importance of good posture in reducing musculoskeletal discomfort among older adults participating in yoga programs (Yao et al., 2023). When you maintain a neutral spine and align your body correctly, you distribute the workload evenly, reducing the risk of discomfort or overexertion.

Optimizing Breath Control

The breath is a fundamental aspect of yoga, influencing physical and mental health. Proper posture facilitates optimal breath control during chair yoga. When your spine is aligned, the respiratory muscles can function efficiently, allowing deep and mindful breathing. This synchronized connection between posture and breath enhances the meditative aspects of chair yoga, promoting relaxation and a heightened sense of presence (aka "awareness").

Enhancing Circulation and Vitality

Maintaining proper posture in chair yoga supports healthy circulation throughout the body. When your spine is aligned, blood flow is unimpeded, delivering essential nutrients and oxygen to various tissues and organs. Another study also suggests that proper posture in yoga helps improve cardiovascular function, enhancing mobility and fitness. (Bharshankar et al., 2003). This improved circulation bolsters vitality, instilling a sense of rejuvenation and energy. Proper posture ensures that the benefits of chair yoga extend beyond the physical, promoting overall vitality and wellness.

Preventing Injuries

One of the primary goals of chair yoga is to provide a safe and accessible form of exercise, especially for seniors or individuals with mobility concerns. Proper posture is a key factor in injury prevention. By aligning your body correctly, you reduce the risk of strains, sprains, or other injuries from improper movement. Emphasizing the importance of correct posture instills a mindful and intentional approach to the practice of chair yoga, minimizing the likelihood of accidents.

Facilitating Mind-Body Connection

Chair yoga is not just a physical practice; it encompasses the integration of mind and body. Proper posture serves as a bridge between the physical and mental aspects of the practice. You create a foundation for mindfulness and introspection when your body is aligned. This mind-body connection deepens the therapeutic benefits of chair yoga, promoting a holistic approach to your better self.

Cultivating Mindful Awareness

Conscious awareness of your body and alignment is integral to chair yoga. Proper posture brings mindful awareness as you engage with each pose. You develop a deeper connection to the present moment by paying attention to your body's alignment. This mindful awareness extends beyond your chair yoga practice, influencing your posture in daily activities and improving overall postural health.

To summarize, proper/correct posture is not merely a technical aspect of chair yoga but a foundational principle that shapes the entire practice. By prioritizing alignment, you unlock the full potential of each pose, ensuring a safe, comfortable, and transformative experience.

Tips for Consistent Practice

Starting a chair yoga journey is an empowering decision. Being consistent with your chair yoga practice is critical to reaping its maximum benefits. Here are practical tips to help you establish and maintain a routine that aligns with your lifestyle and goals.

Create a Dedicated Space: As mentioned earlier in this chapter, transforming a corner of your home into a sanctuary for chair yoga brings many benefits. Clear the space of distractions, and add elements that inspire tranquility, such as plants or soft lighting. A dedicated space enhances focus and serves as a visual cue to prioritize your practice. Most people will be doing these poses <u>inside</u> the home...

Set Realistic Goals: Establishing realistic goals is imperative for sustaining motivation. Consider your current schedule and commitments, then set achievable objectives for your chair yoga practice. Whether committing to three sessions a week or gradually progressing through poses, realistic goals create a sense of accomplishment.

Establish a Routine: Consistency thrives on routine. Integrate chair yoga seamlessly into your daily life by establishing a fixed practice time. Whether it is a morning stretch to invigorate your day or an evening ritual for relaxation, adhering to a routine makes chair yoga a natural and non-negotiable part of your schedule. Some people will do a 10-minute session every morning as their coffee gets ready while they utilize this time more mindfully. Turn on the coffee machine and use that time to stretch and do some chair yoga. Incorporating it into another habit makes it easier to be consistent.

Use Reminders and Alarms: Leverage the convenience of technology to stay on track. Set gentle reminders on your phone or use alarms to prompt your chair yoga practice. These reminders serve as gentle nudges, ensuring you do not inadvertently overlook your commitment to self-care.

Find a Chair Yoga Buddy: Enlisting a friend or family member as your chair yoga buddy can add a delightful social aspect to your practice. Share your goals, progress, and experiences with your buddy. Consider attending virtual classes together or discussing your chair yoga journey regularly. Mutual support can significantly enhance consistency.

Keep It Short and Simple: Recognize that consistency is more achievable when your practice aligns with your lifestyle. If time constraints are a concern, aim for shorter sessions. Even a 10-to 15-minute chair yoga routine can be remarkably effective. Prioritizing quality over quantity ensures that your practice remains sustainable.

Explore Online Resources: Embrace the wealth of online resources available for chair yoga. Explore virtual classes, instructional videos, or mobile apps that cater to your preferences. Having a diverse range of resources allows you to customize your practice based on your mood, energy levels, or specific focus areas.

Track Your Progress: Create a chair yoga journal or utilize a tracking app to document your progress. Regularly jotting down your experiences, achievements, and insights can be motivating. Reflect on how each session makes you feel, and celebrate the milestones in your chair yoga journey. Tracking progress reinforces the positive impact of your consistent practice.

Remember, consistency is about building a sustainable habit rather than aiming for perfection. Gradually incorporating these tips into your routine will contribute to the longevity of your chair yoga practice, ensuring it becomes an integral and enjoyable aspect of your overall well-being.

Final Words

As we explore ways to create a conducive space and foster consistency in your chair yoga practice, let us reflect on the wisdom shared in our opening quote: "Exercise not only changes your body, it changes your mind, your attitude, and your mood." This sentiment encapsulates the transformative potential of chair yoga, not just as a physical exercise but as a holistic practice that positively impacts your entire well-being (Body-Mind Connection).

Key Takeaways

Sanctuary of Serenity: By creating a dedicated space for chair yoga, you've crafted a personal sanctuary infused with tranquility. This space becomes a haven where the stresses of the outside world melt away, allowing you to immerse yourself fully in the transformative practice of chair yoga.

Visual Cues for Prioritization: The intentional setup of your practice area serves as a visual cue, signaling the importance of prioritizing self-care. The absence of distractions and the inclusion of elements that inspire calmness reinforce the commitment to making chair yoga an integral part of your daily routine.

Consistent Reminder: Your dedicated space consistently reminds you of your commitment to well-being. Every time you step into this space, it becomes a reaffirmation of the positive changes you nurture within yourself—physically, mentally, and emotionally.

As we transition to the next chapter, we will explore the fundamental poses forming chair yoga's heart. These poses are not mere exercises but gateways to enhanced flexibility, strength, and holistic well-being. Join us in exploring fundamental chair yoga poses that empower and uplift you in every session.

Step #3: Fundamental Poses

"Your body will be around a lot longer than that expensive handbag. Invest in yourself." — Unknown.

Remember this quote? Well, this chapter is all about investing in yourself, and we're starting with the basics of chair yoga poses. It's like laying the foundation for a sturdy house, setting you up for success in chair yoga, no matter your skill level.

Our goal here is simple — we want to give you the lowdown on the basic chair yoga poses. These poses aren't meant to be tricky; they're like the ABCs of chair yoga. By understanding these fundamentals, you'll be well-prepared to tackle more advanced stuff. The takeaway? We want to empower you, giving you the tools to embrace your chair yoga journey and boost your confidence, mobility, balance, and longevity.

Warm-up Exercises

Warm-up exercises are preliminary activities designed to prepare the body for more intense physical activity. These exercises serve as a transition from a state of rest to increased levels of activity, gradually raising the heart rate and warming the muscles. (American Heart Association, 2014).

Why exercise warm-ups are important

Warm-up exercises help prepare the body for more strenuous activities. These exercises lead to blood vessel dilation, reduced heart load, and boosted circulation, ensuring the muscles receive a heightened blood and oxygen supply. Other benefits include:

• Increasing body temperature during warm-ups enhances muscle elasticity, supporting better flexibility.

• Warm-ups activate mechanisms for cooling, such as sweating, to prevent the body from overheating during intense exercise.

• Hormones released during warm-ups help convert fatty acids and carbohydrates into energy, ensuring an energy-efficient workout.

Warm-up Exercises for the Upper Body

This section will guide you through simple yet effective warm-up exercises tailored for seated practice. Scan the QR Code to access the video demonstration with model Corina. Don't worry, these exercises are all senior friendly!

Arm Circles

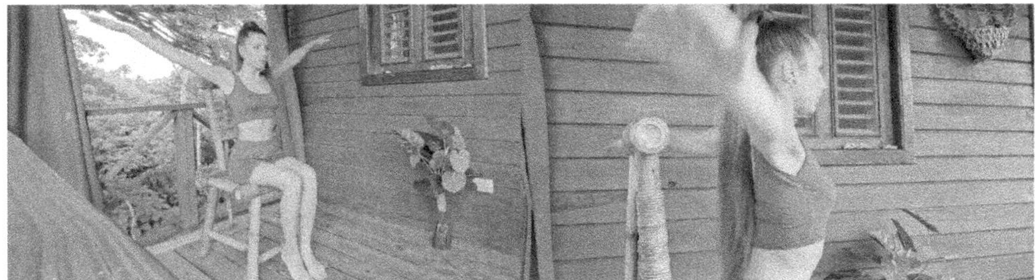

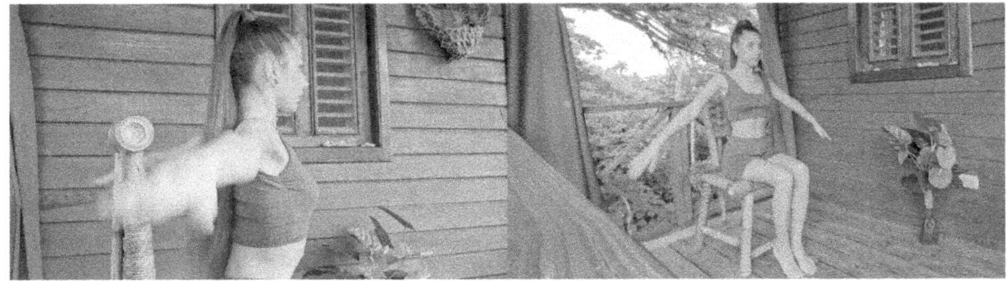

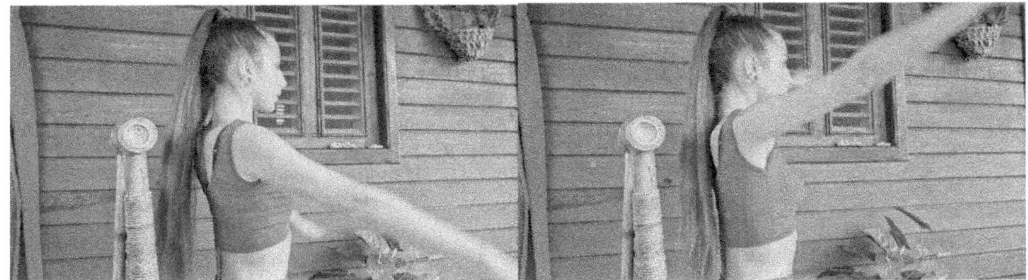

https://youtu.be/pxjOMZNaPB8

• Sit comfortably in a chair with your back straight and shoulders relaxed.

• Extend your arms laterally at shoulder height.

• Begin making circular motions with your arms, moving them forward for 10-15 rotations. You can make small, medium, or large circles depending on your allowed range of motion.

• Reverse the direction, circling your arms backward for another 10-15 rotations.

• Feel the subtle stretch in your shoulders and upper arms while performing these circular motions.

Shoulder Stretch

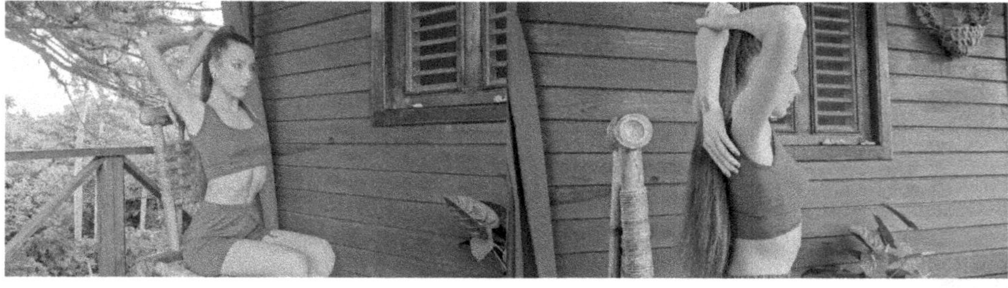

https://youtu.be/uIyvwpeR-tU

- Sit in a chair while keeping your spine straight and shoulders relaxed.
- Lift one arm straight up and bend the elbow, reaching your hand down your back.
- With your opposite hand, gently hold your bent elbow.
- Feel the stretch along the triceps and the back of the arm.
- Hold for 15-20 seconds and switch to the other arm.

Shoulder Rolls

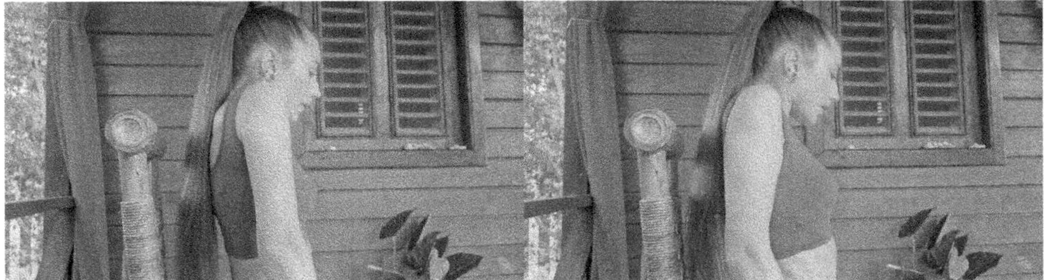

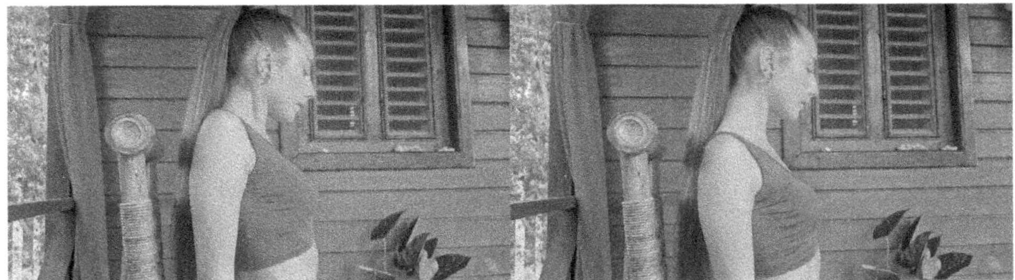

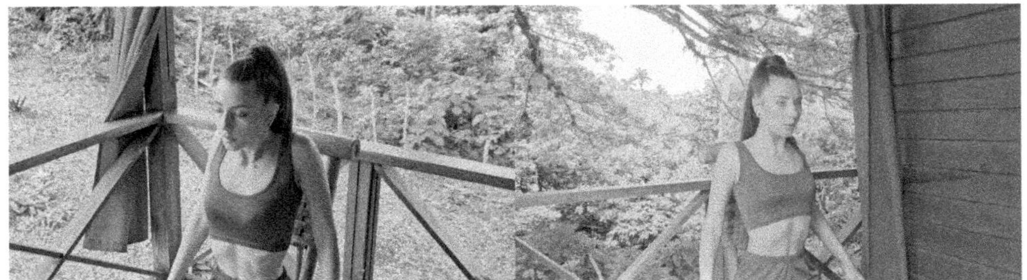

https://youtu.be/tlPCHANbBug

- Sit with an erect posture and relax your arms by your sides.
- Inhale as you lift your shoulders towards your ears.
- Exhale as you roll your shoulders back and down in a circular motion.
- Repeat this movement for 10-15 rotations, then reverse the direction for another 10-15.
- Feel the release of tension in your shoulders and upper back.

Integrate these upper body warm-up exercises into your chair yoga routine to prep your body for the upcoming fundamental poses. Regularly practicing these warm-ups will not only boost your flexibility and range of motion but also result in a safer and more enjoyable chair yoga experience.

Gentle Neck and Shoulder Stretches

After warming up your upper body, the next step in your chair yoga practice is to focus on gentle neck and shoulder stretches. These stretches are designed to alleviate tension, improve flexibility, and promote relaxation while comfortably seated in your chair. Follow the step-by-step instructions for each stretch to enhance your well-being and create a soothing foundation for the chair yoga poses.

Lateral Neck Flexion

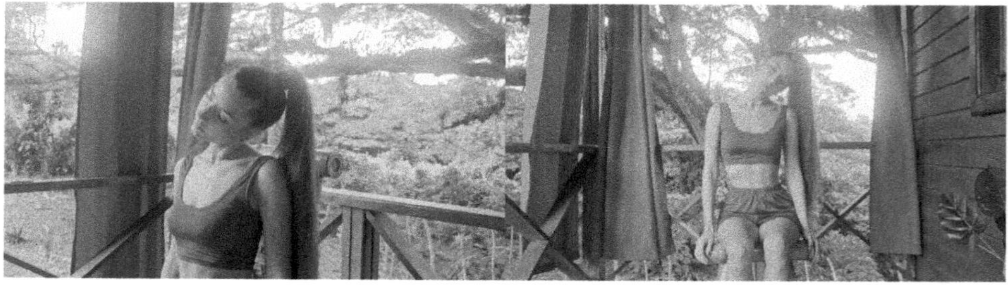

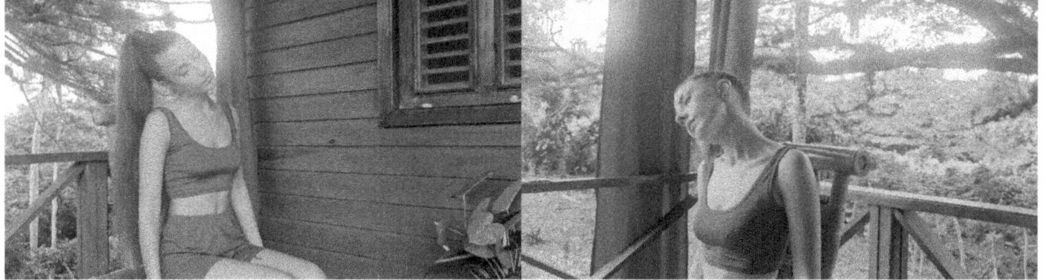

https://youtu.be/XTG1wVoN1zU

- Sit with an upright posture and shoulders relaxed.
- Tilt your head to one side, bringing your ear towards your shoulder.
- Hold for 15-20 seconds, feeling the stretch along the side of your neck.
- Repeat on the other side.
- Continue alternating sides for a total of 2-3 repetitions.

Neck Flexion

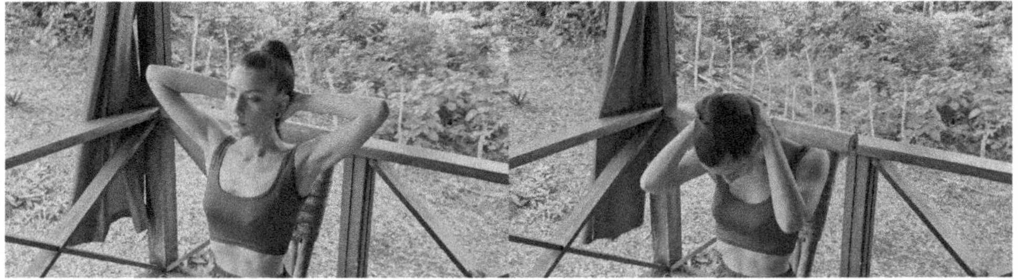

https://youtu.be/xCpvNj9-cro

• Sit comfortably in the chair with your feet flat on the floor and hands behind your head.

• Inhale and engage your core as you curl your head over your shoulders.

• Continue rolling your neck forward like you are bringing your chin closer to the chest.

• Reach the end of your available range of motion, and you must feel a gentle stretch on the back of your neck.

• Exhale and slowly roll your head towards the back of the chair until it is straight over your shoulders, repeating the exercise 2-3 more times.

• If comfortable, incorporate a gentle lean back after sitting straight up, maintaining stability.

• Focus on controlled movements and breath awareness throughout.

Neck Extension

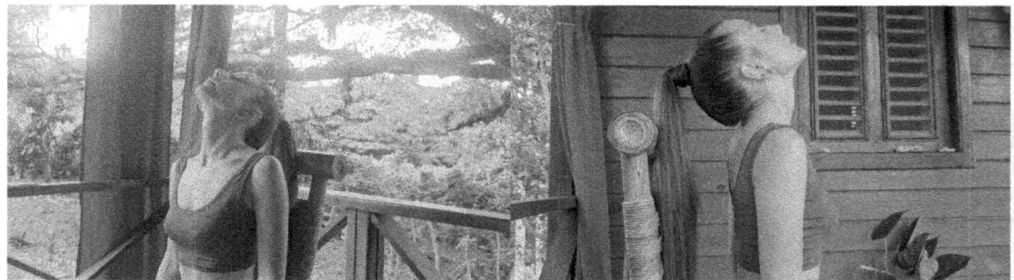

https://youtu.be/KniZQqIfNK8

- Sit with a straight spine and shoulders relaxed.
- Slowly tilt your head backward, bringing your chin towards the ceiling.
- Hold the stretch for 15-20 seconds, feeling the gentle elongation along the front of your neck.
- Return your head to a neutral position.

Neck Rotation

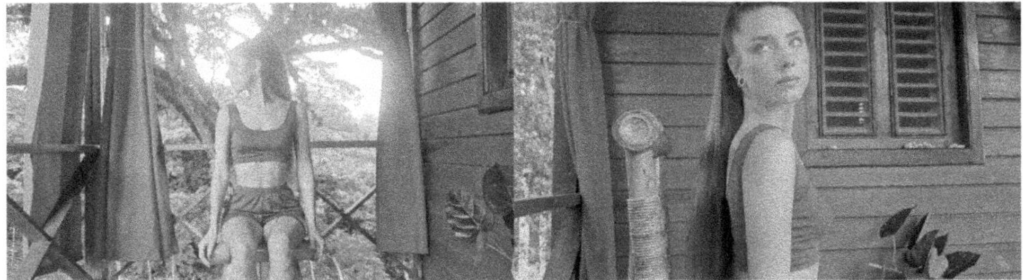

https://youtu.be/zUMFU1noGjo

- Sit tall and slowly turn your head to one side, bringing your chin towards your shoulder.
- Hold the stretch for 15-20 seconds, feeling the release in the neck and upper spine.

- Repeat on the other side.
- Continue alternating sides for a total of 2-3 repetitions.

Chin Movements

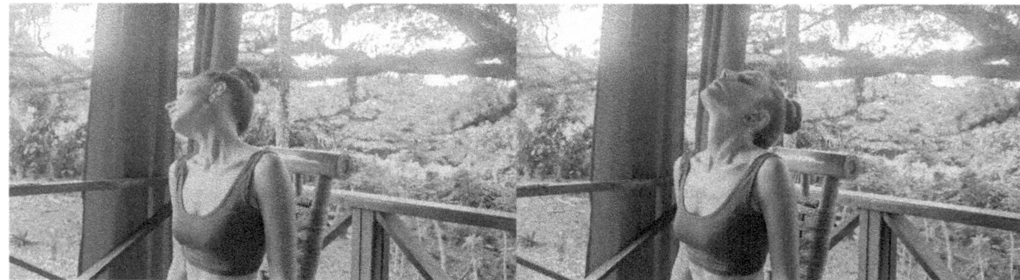

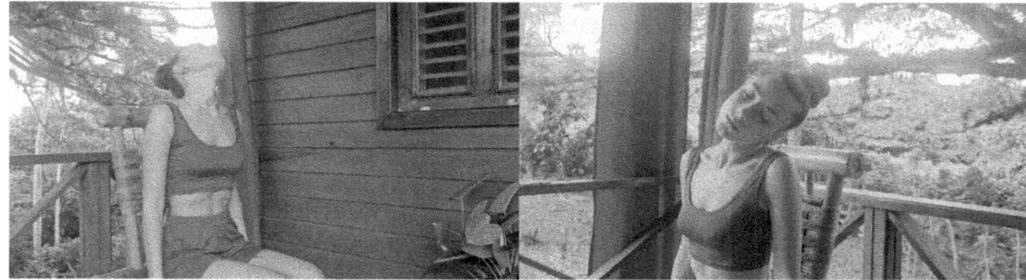

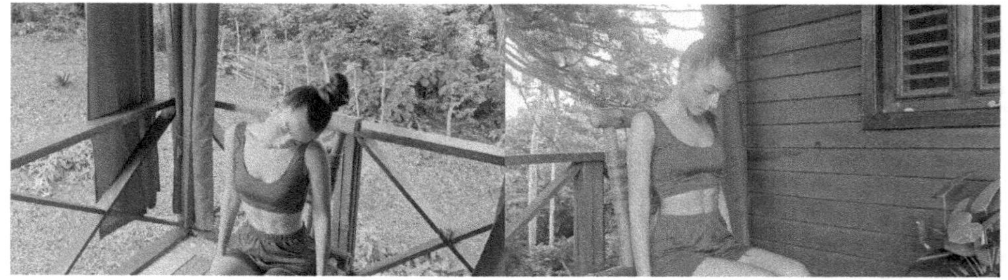

https://youtu.be/zgGXzfUfYyw

- Sit comfortably and tilt your head to one side, bringing your ear towards your shoulder.
- Slowly draw circles with your chin, moving it gently in one direction.
- After 5-10 rotations, reverse the direction of the circles.
- Feel the subtle stretch and improved range of motion in your neck.

Shoulder Raises

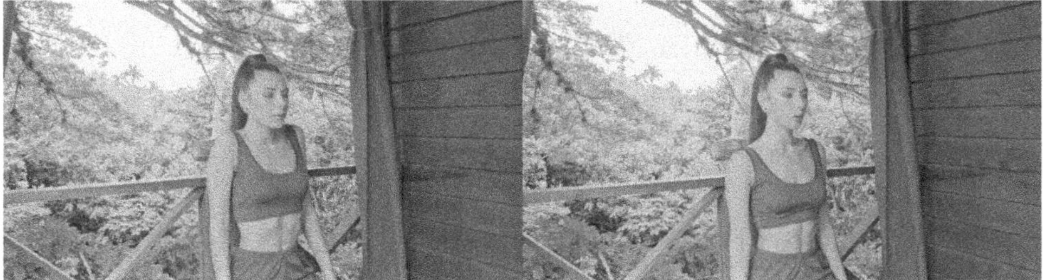

https://youtu.be/zTb9t5svFDQ

- Sit comfortably and relax your arms by your sides.
- Inhale as you lift both shoulders towards your ears.
- Exhale as you lower your shoulders back down.
- Repeat for 10-15 repetitions, focusing on the gentle movement and relaxation of your shoulder muscles.

Adding these gentle neck and shoulder stretches into your chair yoga routine promotes flexibility, releases tension, and enhances overall health. These seated stretches are perfect for relaxation and fostering a deeper connection with your body during your chair yoga practice.

. . .

Seated Twists for Improved Spinal Mobility

Enhancing spinal mobility is key in chair yoga as it improves overall flexibility. Seated twists are excellent for gently engaging and mobilizing the spine while maintaining a seated position. The following instructions will guide you through three versions of seated twists, allowing you to experience the benefits of improved spinal mobility in your chair yoga practice.

Seated Twist with Gentle Hold

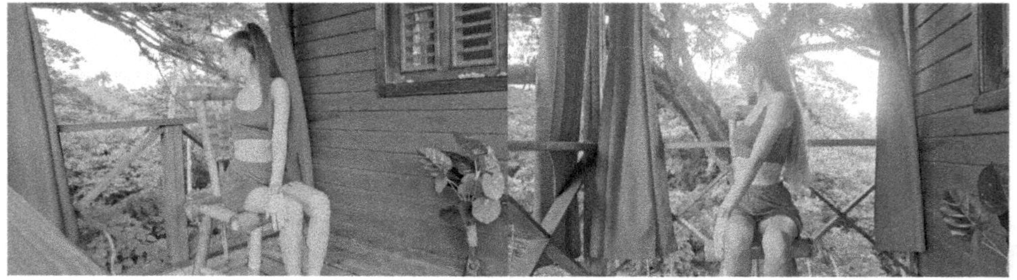

https://youtu.be/LG5SeNQU6jE

- Sit comfortably with a straight spine and both feet flat on the floor.
- Inhale and lengthen your spine, then exhale as you gently twist to one side.
- Place one hand on the opposite knee and the other on the back of your chair.
- Hold the twist for 15-20 seconds, feeling the gentle stretch along your spine.
- Inhale back to the center and repeat on the other side.
- Continue alternating sides for 2-3 repetitions.

Chair Twist with Arm Reach

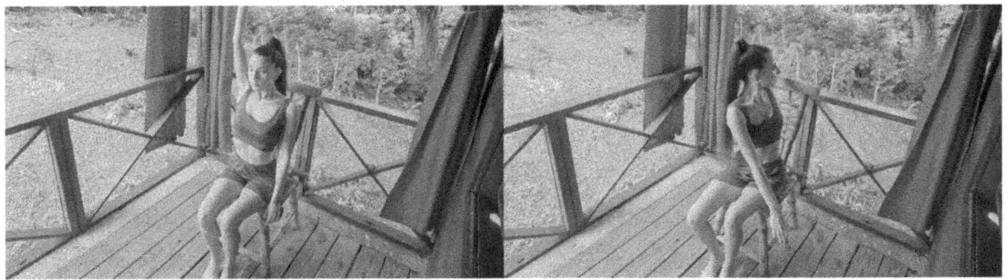

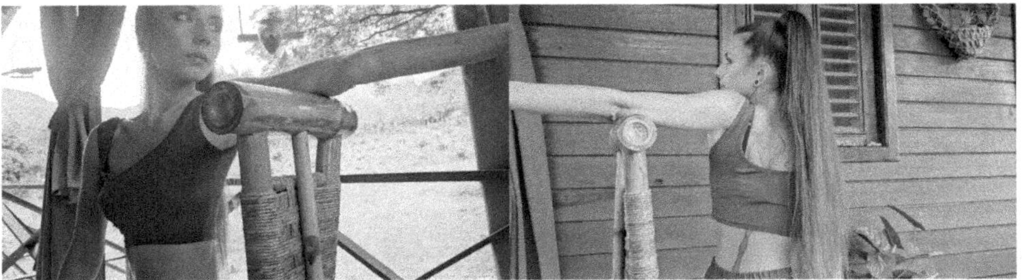

https://youtu.be/XJhxPKDbXoI

- Sit on a chair with your back straight and feet flat on the floor or on the ground if performing outside.

- Inhale, lift one arm towards the ceiling or the sky and exhale as you twist towards the opposite side.

- Place your lifted hand on the outside of the opposite thigh or knee.

- Extend your opposite arm behind you, resting it on the back of the chair.

- Hold the twist for 15-20 seconds, feeling the elongation of your spine.

- Inhale back to the center and repeat on the other side.
- Alternate sides for 2-3 repetitions.

Seated Twist Cat-Cow Variation

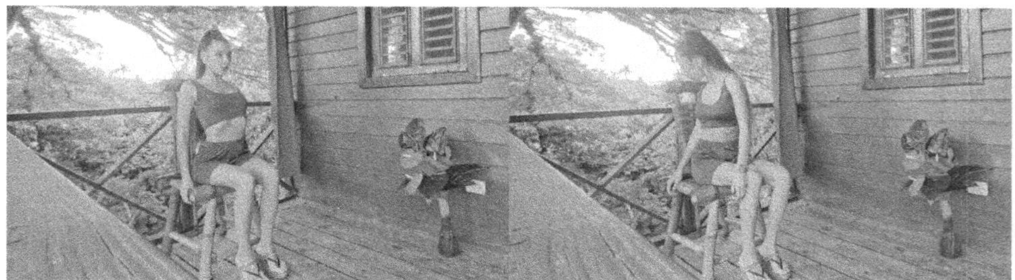

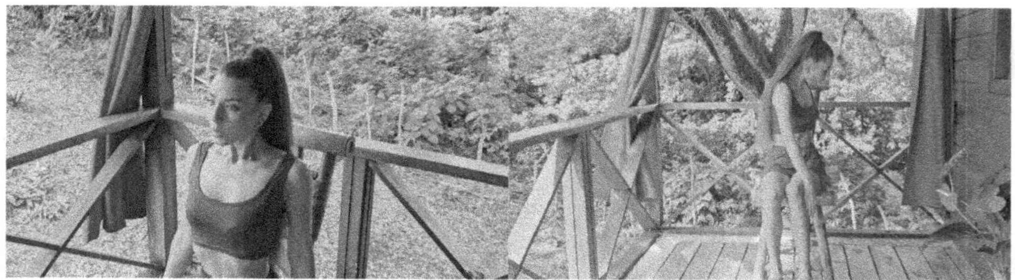

https://youtu.be/ozj2dc8InF8

- Sit comfortably with an upright posture.
- Inhale as you lengthen your spine and engage your core.
- Exhale and twist to one side, bringing your opposite hand to the outside of your knee.
- Inhale back to the center, exhale as you turn to the other side.

- Coordinate the movement with your breath, flowing smoothly between twists.
- Repeat for 1-2 minutes, gradually increasing the range of motion.

Integrate these easy seated twists into your chair yoga routine to improve spinal mobility, alleviate stiffness, and promote a healthier, more flexible spine. These twists are accessible and effective, making them perfect for seniors seeking to improve their health through chair yoga.

Effective Arm and Hand Movements

Arm and hand movements are another important component of chair yoga, resulting in overall flexibility and relieving tension in the upper body. The following hand and arm stretches provide a simple yet effective way to enhance mobility, reduce stiffness, and promote relaxation while seated. (*Exercises for Pain Free Hands*, 2013)

Claw Stretch

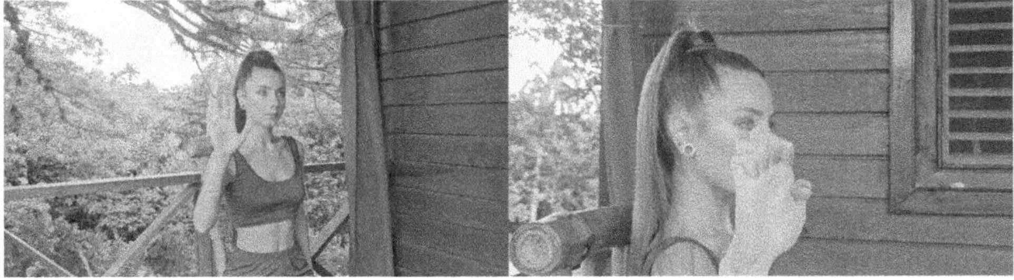

https://youtu.be/pFAC5IXECEY

- Sit comfortably with a straight spine and relax your shoulders.
- Make a "claw" with your hand
- Hold the stretch for 10-15 seconds, feeling the opening and stretch in your hand and fingers.

• Release and repeat for 2-3 repetitions, gently alternating between hands.

Grip Strengthening

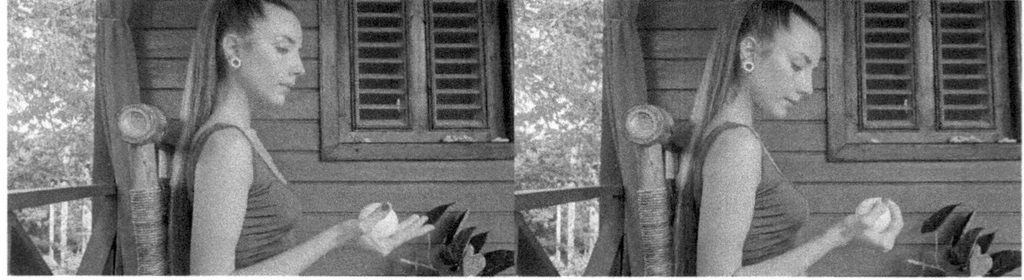

https://youtu.be/wu6zou3AFpc

• Sit well and place a small, soft, or stress ball in one hand.

• Squeeze the ball, engaging your hand muscles.

• Hold the squeeze for a few seconds, then release.

• Repeat the squeeze-and-release motion for 10-15 repetitions on each hand.

Finger Stretch

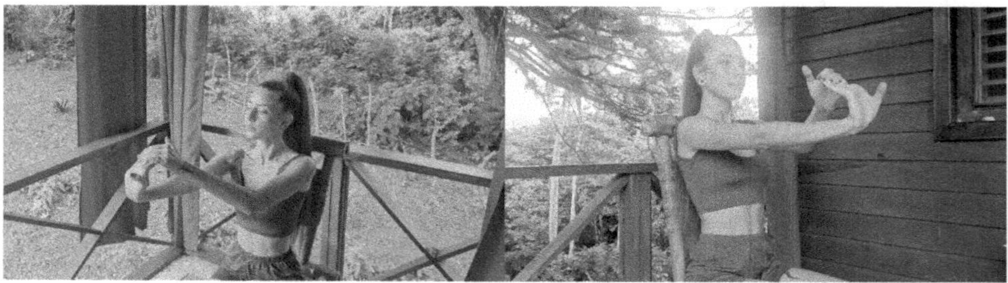

https://youtu.be/h67iVKxT_js

- Sit comfortably and extend your arm forward at shoulder height.
- With your opposite hand, gently push each finger backward, stretching the fingers and the palm.
- Hold the stretch for fifteen to thirty seconds and release.
- Repeat, on the other hand, alternating for 2-3 repetitions.
- This stretch promotes flexibility and alleviates tension in the fingers.

Wrist Circles

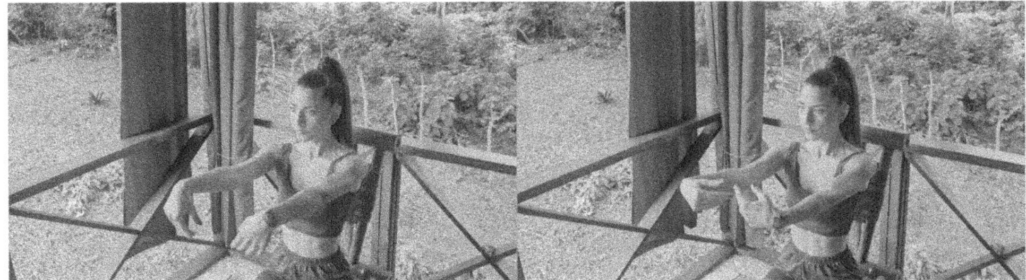

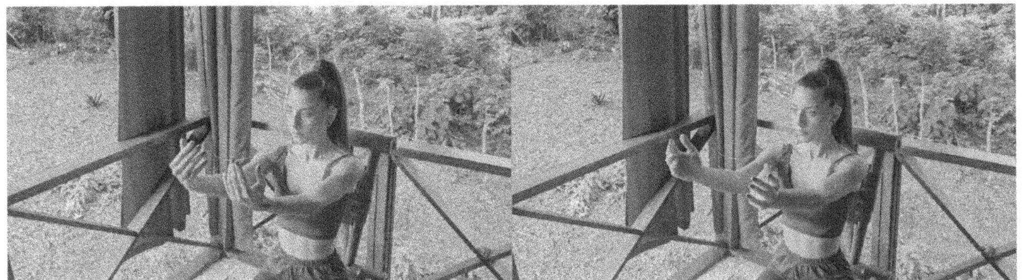

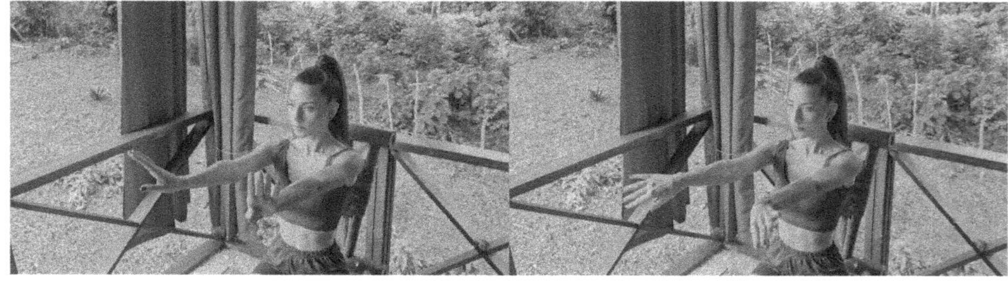

https://youtu.be/VZFOMEooQJw

- Sit with your back straight and shoulders relaxed.
- Extend your arms forward and rotate your wrists in a circular motion.
- Perform 10-15 rotations in one direction, then reverse for another 10-15 rotations.
- Wrist circles help improve mobility and reduce stiffness in the wrists and forearms.

Forearm Stretch

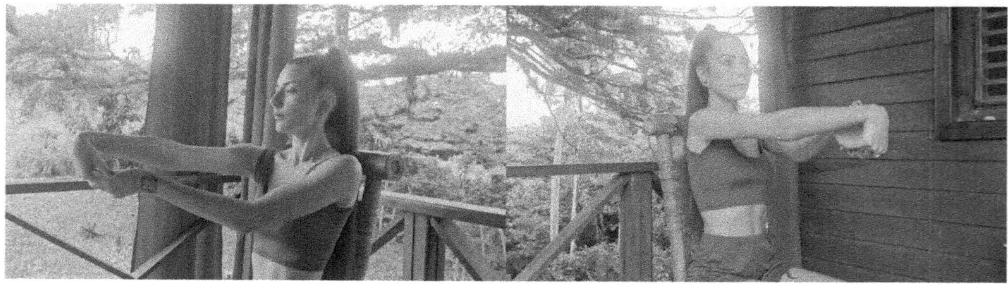

https://youtu.be/HsfZIbXY-tY

- Sit tall and extend one arm forward with your palm facing down.
- Use your opposite hand to gently press down on the fingers of the outstretched hand.
- Feel the stretch along the top of the forearm.
- Hold for 15-20 seconds and switch to the other arm.
- Repeat for 2-3 repetitions on each side.

Adding these hand and arm movements into your chair yoga routine promotes flexibility, strengthens hand muscles, and alleviates tension. These stretches are simple yet effective, providing a mindful and accessible approach to improving the well-being of your hands and arms while seated.

Strengthening the Core While Seated

Chair yoga offers a unique and accessible way to strengthen the core muscles while remaining comfortably seated. Engaging the core is vital for stability, balance, and overall strength. This section overviews how chair yoga targets different core muscles and encourages you to actively engage with simple motions to feel each area. (*How to Engage Your Core: Steps, Muscles Worked, and More*, 2022)

Deep Abdominal Muscles (Transverse Abdominis)

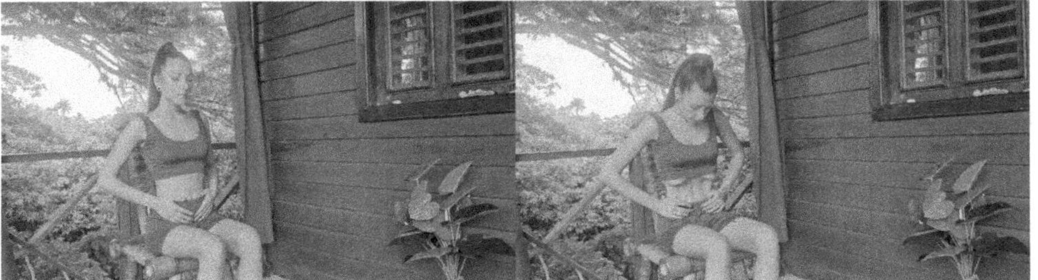

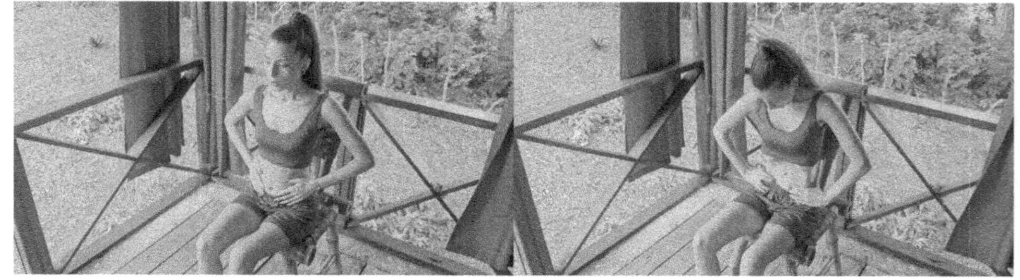

https://youtu.be/112Qrf25qtc

- Sit comfortably and place your hands on your lower abdomen.
- Inhale deeply and expand your abdomen.
- Exhale completely, drawing your navel towards your spine.
- Feel the contraction in the deep abdominal muscles. Repeat for 5-10 breaths.

Rectus Abdominis (Upper Abdominals)

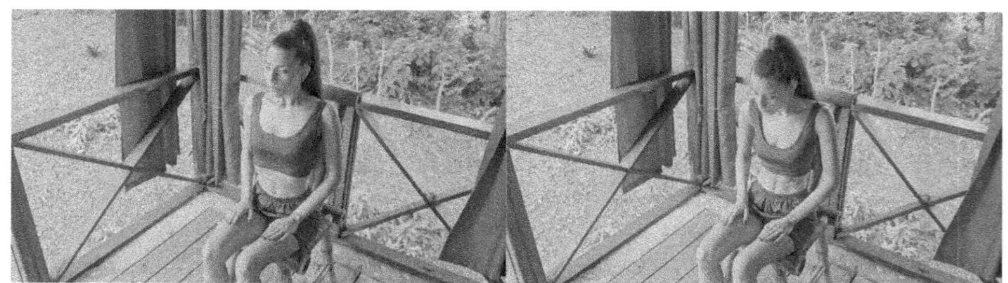

https://youtu.be/4UVb_wAbdvY

• Sit with an upright posture and place your hands on your thighs.

• Inhale and lift your chest slightly while maintaining a straight spine.

• Exhale and engage your upper abdominal muscles, bringing your chest towards your thighs.

• Feel the contraction in the upper abdominal area. Repeat for 5-10 breaths.

Obliques (Side Abdominals)

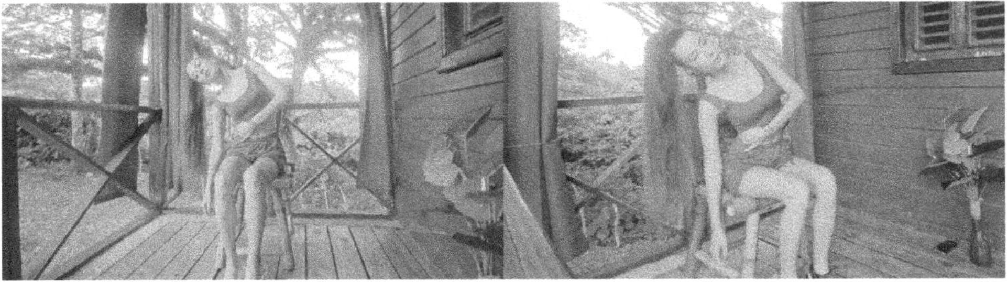

https://youtu.be/2FEfjE7joLY

• Sit tall and place one hand on the opposite side of your waist.

• Inhale deeply, and as you exhale, gently lean to the side, engaging the oblique muscles.

• Feel the stretch on one side and the contraction on the other. Inhale back to the center and repeat on the opposite side.

Lower Back (Erector Spinae)

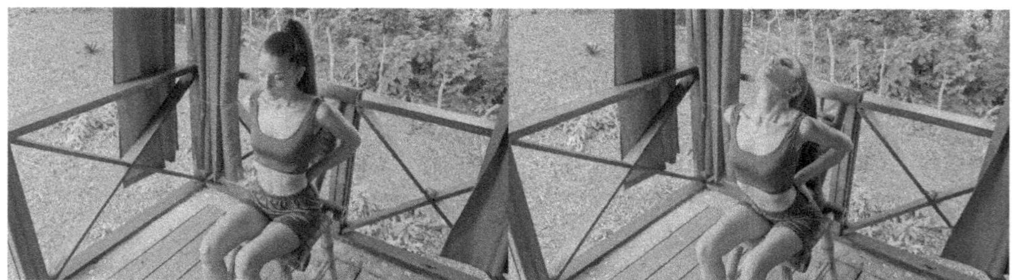

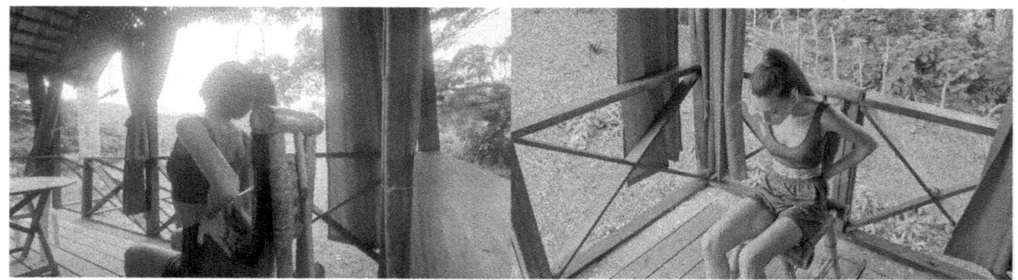

https://youtu.be/o6zp7aa8ALY

• Sit with a straight spine and your hands on your lower back.

• Inhale, lengthening your spine, and gently arch your back.

• Exhale, engaging your lower back muscles, and round your spine.

• Feel the stretch and contraction along the lower back. Repeat for 5-10 breaths.

Pelvic Floor Muscles

- Sit comfortably and focus on the muscles in your pelvic floor.
- Inhale and engage the muscles as if you were stopping the urine flow.
- Exhale and release. Repeat this gentle contraction and release for 5-10 breaths.

By actively engaging with these simple motions, you can heighten your awareness of different core muscles. Regular practice of chair yoga will not only strengthen these core muscles but also lead to improved posture and mobility. As you progress through your chair yoga routine, pay attention to the subtle engagement of these core muscles, creating a deeper connection with your body and enhancing your holistic wellness.

Chair Yoga Poses for Better Leg Flexibility

Improving leg flexibility is imperative for mobility and overall health. Chair yoga provides an excellent opportunity to enhance leg flexibility while maintaining a seated position. The following chair yoga poses focus on basic aspects of leg flexibility, making them accessible for practitioners of all levels. Incorporate these poses into your routine to experience increased flexibility and improved leg mobility.

Seated Forward Bend

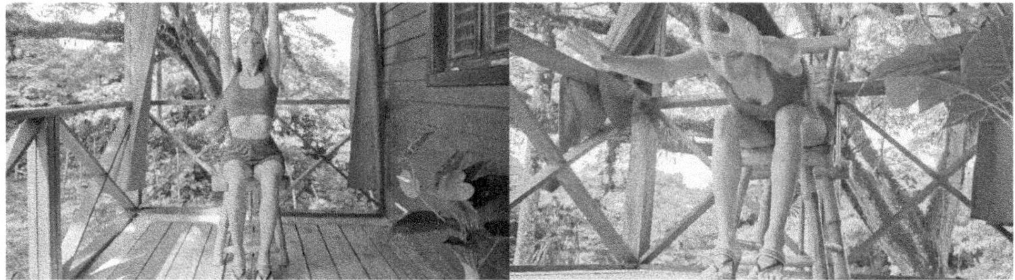

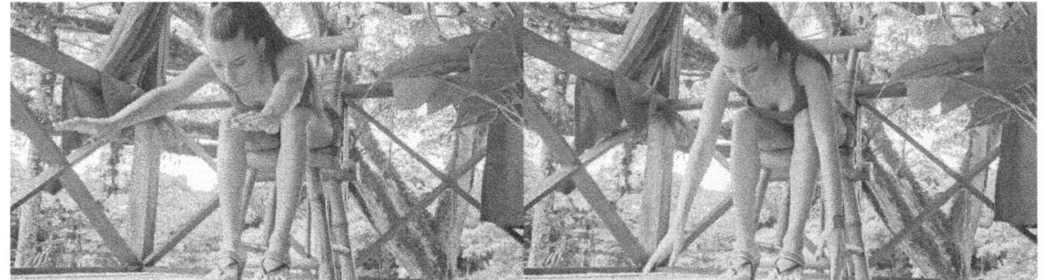

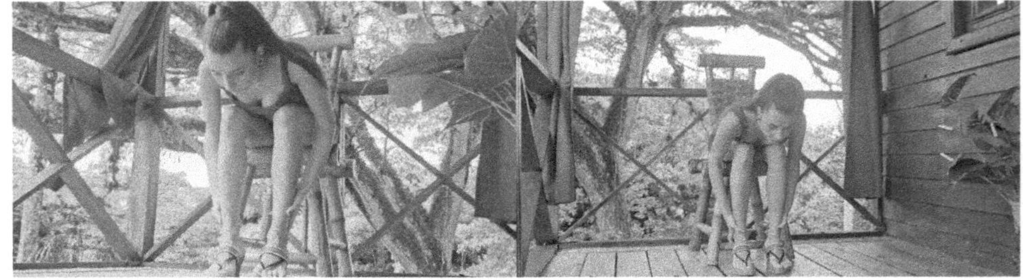

https://youtu.be/GiWmqFrqMCo

- Sit at the front edge of a chair with your feet flat on the floor or on the ground if performing these outside.
- Inhale deeply, elongating your spine, and raise your arms overhead. You can also keep them on your thighs.
- Exhale as you hinge at your hips, extending your hands toward your feet.
- If possible, grasp your shins or ankles. If not, let your hands rest on your knees.
- Hold the stretch for 15-20 seconds, feeling the gentle elongation along your hamstrings and lower back.
- Inhale as you return to an upright position.

Chair Pigeon Pose

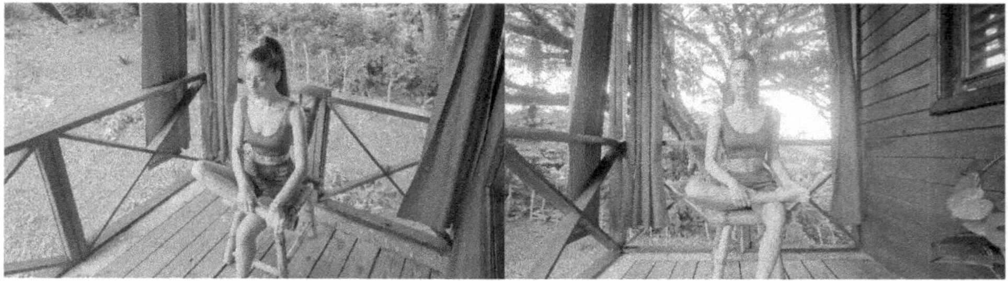

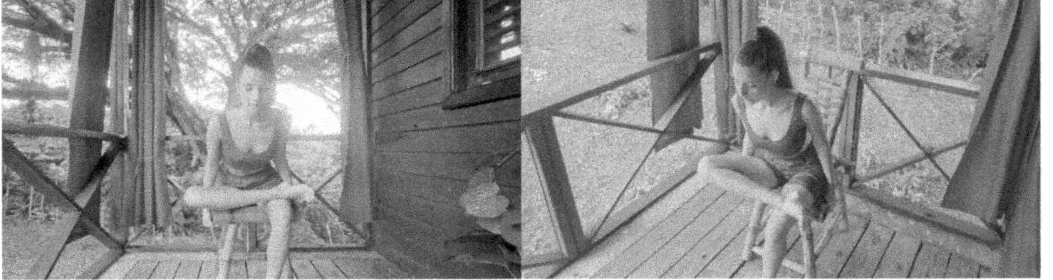

https://youtu.be/i1PzmszWml8

- Sit tall with your feet flat on the floor.
- Lift your right foot and place the outer edge on your left thigh, creating a figure-four shape.
- Flex your right foot to protect the knee and maintain proper alignment.
- If comfortable, hinge forward at the hips, keeping a straight spine.
- Hold the stretch for 15-20 seconds, feeling the release in your right hip and outer thigh.
- Repeat on the other side.

Chair Warrior II

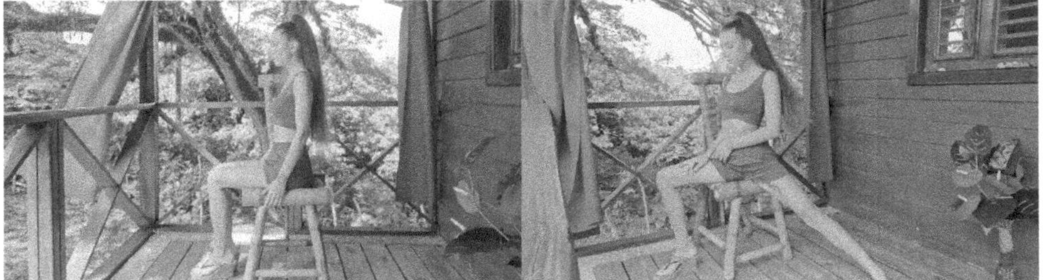

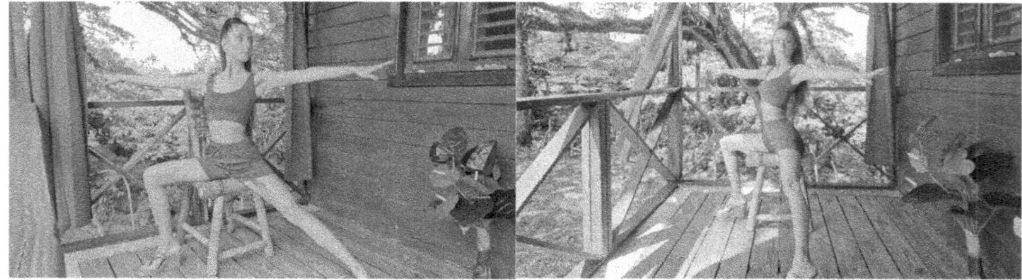

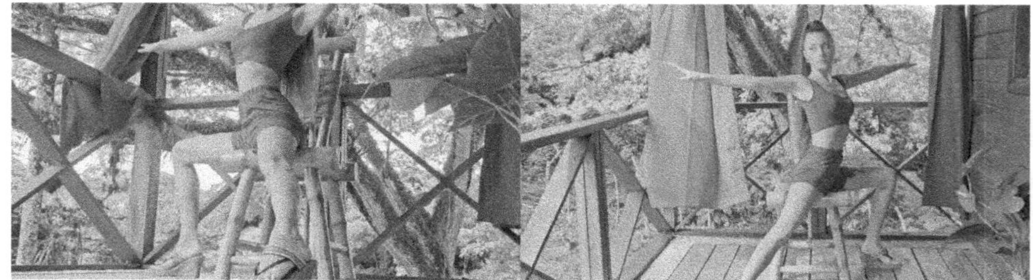

https://youtu.be/Ooc552Z4Voo

- Sit with your right side close to the backrest of the chair.
- Extend your left leg straight to the side and keep your right foot firmly on the floor.
- Rotate your upper body to face the right extending your arms parallel to the floor.
- Hold the position for 15-20 seconds, feeling the stretch along the inner thigh and outer hip.
- Repeat on the other side.

These chair yoga poses gently target various leg muscles, promoting flexibility without straining the joints. Regular practice of these poses will help you gain increased leg flexibility and improved range of motion while reducing the risk of falls. Remember to listen to your body, modify as needed, and gradually progress as your flexibility improves.

. . .

Integrating Mindfulness in Every Pose

Mindfulness is a transformative element that can significantly enhance your chair yoga experience. Bringing awareness to each movement and breath fosters a deeper connection between the mind and body, creating a more enriching and holistic practice. (*Yoga and Meditation*, 2020)

The Importance of Mindfulness in Exercise

- Mindfulness means being fully present and engaged in the current moment, resulting in a heightened awareness of sensations, thoughts, and emotions.
- Integrating mindfulness into exercise enhances the mind-body connection, promoting balance and unity.
- Mindful movement encourages a non-judgmental acceptance of your body's capabilities, creating a positive and compassionate attitude toward yourself.

Advice on Including Mindfulness in Chair Yoga

Start with Breath Awareness: Begin each chair yoga session by bringing attention to your breath. Take time to inhale and exhale deeply, anchoring yourself in the present moment.

Body Scan Technique: During warm-up exercises or stretches, perform a mental body scan. Focus on each part of your body, noticing sensations, tension, or areas of relaxation.

Stay Present in Poses: As you move through chair yoga poses, direct your attention to the sensations in your body. Notice how your muscles engage, where you feel stretches and any areas of tension or release.

Mindful Transitions: Focus on the transitions between poses. Mindfully move from one position to the next, maintaining a smooth and intentional flow.

Use breath as an Anchor: Focus on your breath during challenging poses or moments of discomfort. Use the breath as an anchor to stay present and grounded.

Practice Gratitude: Establish a sense of gratitude for your body and the opportunity to engage in chair yoga. Appreciate the moments of stillness and movement as valuable components of your mental focus.

Mindful Closing: Conclude your chair yoga session with a few moments of reflection and gratitude. Acknowledge the positive impact of mindfulness on your physical and mental state.

By infusing mindfulness into your chair yoga routine, you create a harmonious integration of body and mind. This enhances the physical benefits of exercise and nurtures a sense of inner peace. Embrace mindfulness as an integral part of your chair yoga journey, and you'll discover the transformation it brings to both your overall health and wellness.

. . .

Introduction to Meditation and Breathing Techniques

Yoga and meditation are intertwined practices that share a harmonious relationship, aiming to bring inner peace, mindfulness, and integrity. This section will explore the connection between yoga and meditation and guide you on seamlessly integrating meditation into your chair yoga practice. Additionally, we'll introduce four effective breathing techniques to enhance the meditative aspect of the practice.

Yoga and Meditation: A Synergistic Pairing

Yoga and meditation are inseparable companions, each complementing and deepening the benefits of the other. While yoga involves physical postures and movements to promote flexibility and strength, meditation is the practice of stilling the mind to achieve mental clarity and heightened awareness. Together, they form a holistic approach to wellness, combining the physical and mental dimensions. In chair yoga, the marriage of gentle movements and mindful meditation creates a synergy that enhances the overall experience, revitalizing a sense of balance and tranquility.

Guidance on Including Meditation in Chair Yoga:

Begin with Breath Awareness: Start your chair yoga practice with a few minutes of focused breath awareness. Sit comfortably, close your eyes, and focus on your breath. Observe the natural inhalations and exhalations, allowing the breath to guide you into a state of presence. This simple meditation sets the tone for a mindful and centered practice.

Mindful Body Scan: As discussed earlier, mindfully scanning your body as you move through chair yoga poses can be beneficial. Bring your awareness to different body parts, noting any sensations or tension. This practice encourages a deep connection between your mind and body, fostering mindfulness in motion.

Guided Visualization: Incorporate guided visualizations into your chair yoga routine. During moments of stillness, visualize calming scenes or experiences. Whether it's a peaceful beach, a serene forest, or a favorite place, guided visualizations can enhance the meditative aspect of your practice.

Breathing Techniques for Chair Yoga:

Diaphragmatic Breathing

- Sit comfortably with a straight spine.
- Inhale deeply through your nose, allowing your diaphragm to expand.

• Exhale through pursed lips, sensing the contraction in your abdomen.

• Repeat for several breaths, focusing on your diaphragm's smooth, controlled movement.

Alternate Nostril Breathing (Nadi Shodhana)

• Sit comfortably with an upright spine.

• Seal your right nostril with your right thumb and inhale with your left nostril.

• Next, close your left nostril with your right-hand finger, release the right nostril, and exhale.

• Inhale through the right nostril, seal it and exhale through the left nostril.

• This constitutes one cycle; repeat for several rounds, focusing on the equilibrium of breath.

Ujjayi Breath (Ocean Breath)

• Inhale deeply through your nose.

• Exhale slowly through a slightly constricted throat, creating a gentle, audible sound similar to ocean waves.

• Focus on the rhythm and sound of your breath, promoting a calming effect.

Counted Breath Meditation

• Inhale deeply and silently count to four.

• Hold your breath, counting to four.

• Exhale slowly, counting to four.

• Maintain the exhale and count to four.

• Gradually increase the count as your breath becomes more controlled and steady.

Meditation and breathing techniques seamlessly intertwine with chair yoga, adding a dimension of mindfulness and tranquility to your practice. Incorporating guided meditation and purposeful breathwork enhances the holistic benefits of chair yoga, promoting both physical and mental health. Experiment with these techniques to discover their calming influence on your chair yoga experience, creating a space for relaxation, focus, and self-awareness.

. . .

Final Words

As we conclude this chapter on Chair Yoga Fundamentals, we must reflect on our journey toward improved well-being and flexibility. We began by understanding the significance of warm-up exercises, gradually moving through gentle upper-body stretches, neck and shoulder movements, and effective arm and hand stretches. We explored seated twists for improved spinal mobility and engaged in core-strengthening practices while seated. We discovered accessible chair yoga poses that focus on basic aspects of leg flexibility.

However, it is the integration of mindfulness in every pose that truly elevates our chair yoga practice. By finding awareness and being present in each movement, we enhance the physical benefits and build a deeper connection between the mind and body. As we've discussed, mindfulness is the transformative element that brings a sense of balance and unity to our chair yoga journey.

Key Takeaways

Mind-Body Connection: Chair yoga is not just about physical exercise; it's a holistic practice that nurtures the mind-body connection, promoting balance and unity.

Accessible Flexibility: The beauty of chair yoga lies in its accessibility. Each practice is designed to be inclusive, from warm-up exercises to leg stretches, making it suitable for individuals of all fitness levels.

As we anticipate your continued exploration of chair yoga, the upcoming chapters will highlight more advanced poses, building upon our established foundational elements. Get ready to challenge your body and mind further as we move on to Chapter 4: Mastering Beginner Poses. Embrace the journey and explore chair yoga's profound benefits in enhancing your overall health.

Step #4: Mastering Beginner Poses

"It is health that is real wealth and not pieces of gold and silver." —Gandhi.

In the wise words of Gandhi, health is the true wealth we should cherish. This sentiment forms the guiding principle as we advance further into our chair yoga journey. This chapter, "Step #4: Mastering Beginner Poses," serves as a gateway to the core of this book. Here, we unravel 25 beginner poses, accompanied by guidance that lays the foundation for a safe and effective practice. No complicated jargon, just straightforward instructions to help you seamlessly integrate these poses into your daily routine.

Beginner-Friendly Chair Yoga Poses

Here are 25 beginner-friendly chair yoga poses. We will discuss each pose with detailed step-by-step instructions, making them accessible. Whether new to yoga or seeking gentle exercises, these poses are designed to bring tranquility and flexibility to your daily routine.

1. Seated Mountain Pose

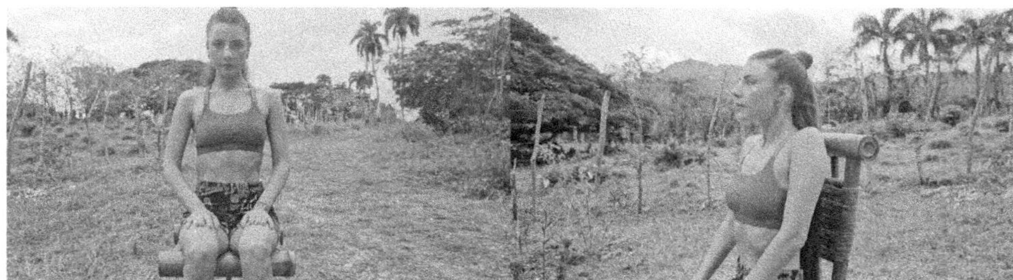

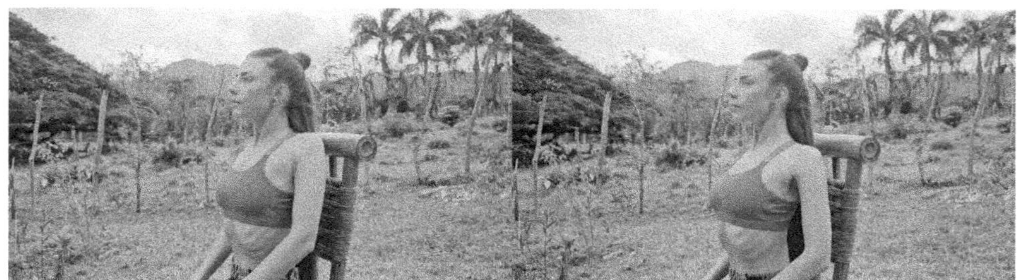

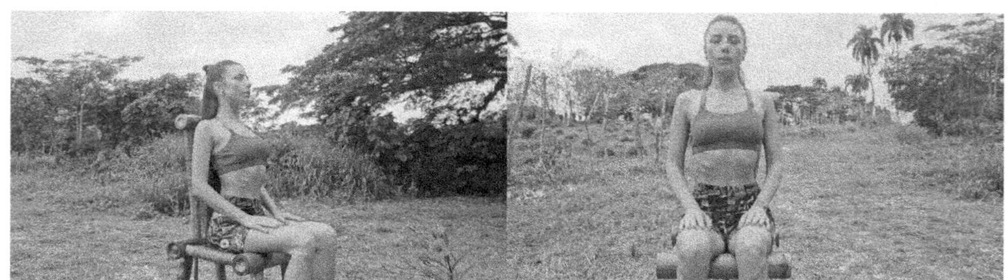

https://youtu.be/w_YPiQDOozc

- Sit comfortably at the front of your chair with your feet flat on the ground.

• Keep your back straight, shoulders relaxed, and hands resting on your thighs.

• Ground your feet evenly, making sure your weight is well-balanced.

• Tighten your tummy slightly to support your lower back without straining.

• Lengthen your spine by lifting the crown of your head.

• Roll your shoulders back and down, opening up your chest.

• Let your arms rest gently on your thighs, palms facing down.

• Keep a slight bend in your elbows to avoid stiffness.

• Take slow, deep breaths through your nose and exhale through your mouth.

• Focus on feeling your chest rise and fall and your ribcage expanding.

• Stay in this pose for 1-3 minutes, adjusting for comfort.

• If you like, close your eyes for a more inward focus.

• To finish, gently open your eyes, release tension, and move slowly to your next pose.

2. Neck Tilts and Turns

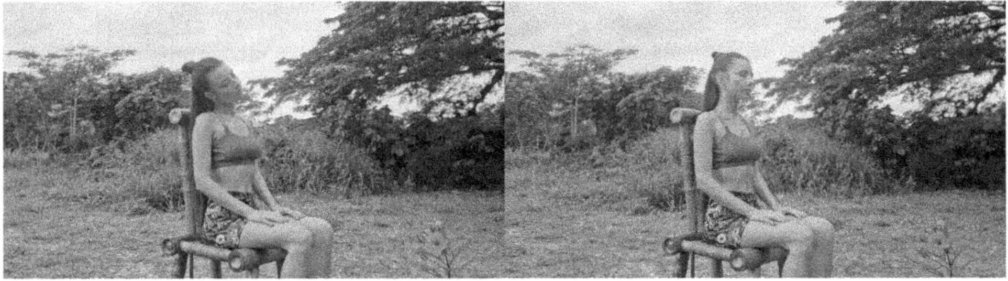

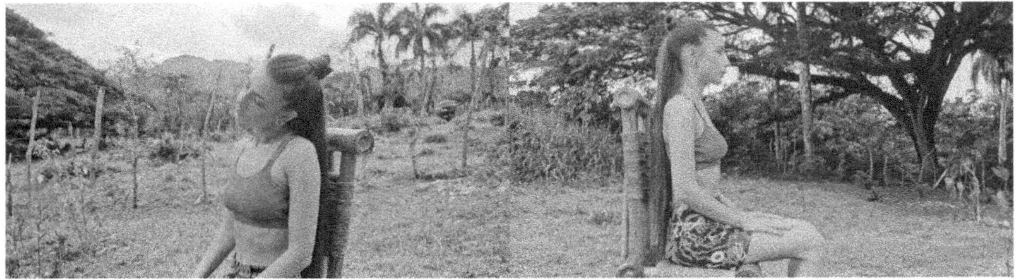

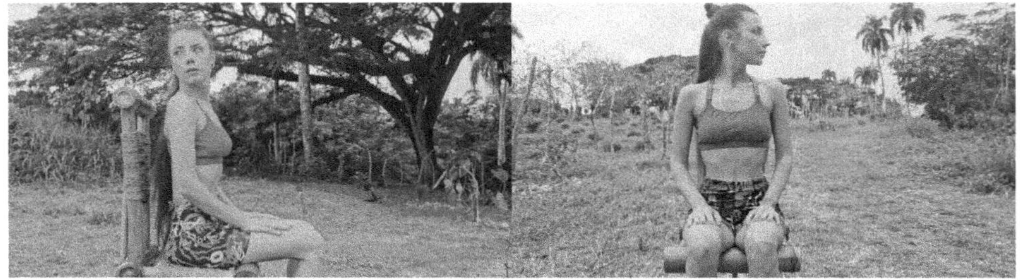

https://youtu.be/VjYIIPEgvUM

- Sit comfortably with a straight back and relaxed shoulders.
- Place your hands on your thighs, palms facing down.
- Slowly tilt your head to the right, bringing your ear towards your shoulder.
- Hold for a few seconds, feeling a gentle stretch on the left side of your neck.
- Return your head to the center.
- Tilt your head to the left, bringing your ear towards your left shoulder.
- Hold for a few seconds, feeling a stretch on the right side of your neck.
- Return your head to the center.
- Gently turn your head to the right, looking over your shoulder.
- Hold for a few seconds, feeling a stretch on the left side of your neck.
- Return your head to the center.
- Turn your head to the left, looking over your left shoulder.
- Hold for a few seconds, feeling a stretch on the right side of your neck.

- Return your head to the center.
- Repeat each tilt and turn 2-3 times, moving slowly.
- If there is any discomfort, reduce the range of motion.
- To finish, return your head to the center and sit, allowing any residual tension to release.

3. Seated Cat-Cow Stretch

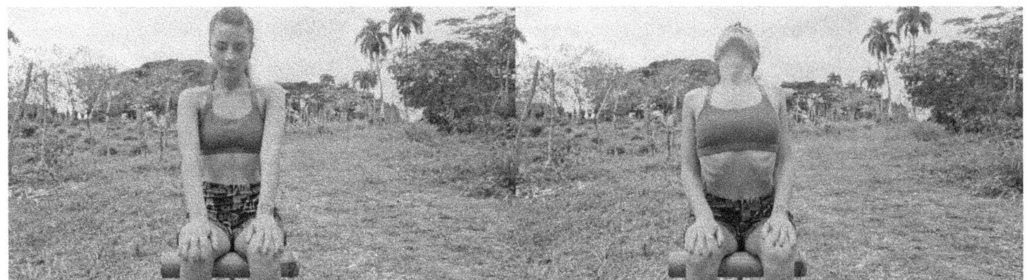

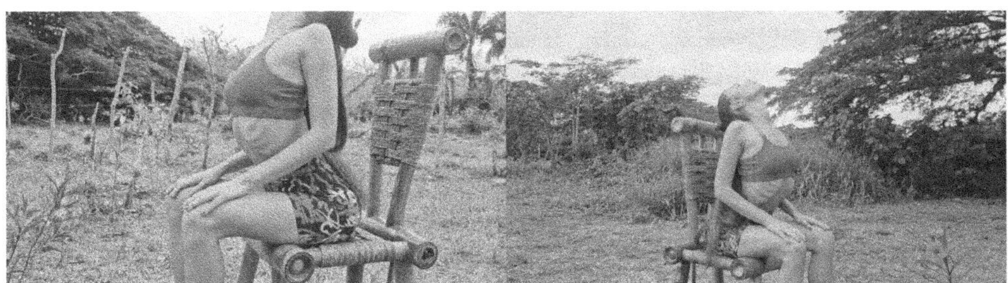

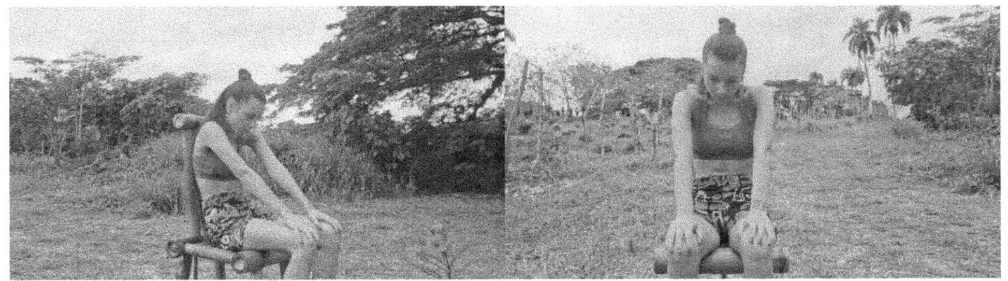

https://youtu.be/4KIaZAWOx6o

- Begin comfortably seated with your feet flat on the ground.
- Place your hands on your knees, keeping your spine straight.
- Inhale slowly, arching your back and lifting your chest towards the ceiling.
- Open your shoulders, allowing your shoulder blades to come together (Cow Pose).
- Exhale gently, rounding your back and tucking your chin towards your chest.
- Feel the stretch along your spine and between your shoulder blades (Cat Pose).
- Inhale, returning to the Cow Pose with an arched back.
- Keep the movement fluid, syncing your breath with the stretch.
- Exhale, moving back to the Cat Pose, rounding your back.
- Continue this gentle rocking motion, flowing between Cat and Cow poses.
- Focus on the movement originating from your pelvis and flowing through your spine.
- Repeat the sequence for about 1-2 minutes, maintaining a smooth and steady pace.
- Be mindful of your breath, inhaling during the Cow Pose and exhaling during the Cat Pose.
- If you experience discomfort, reduce the range of motion and move within your comfort zone.
- To conclude, return to a neutral seated position and take a moment to feel the newfound flexibility and release in your spine.

4. Wrist Circles

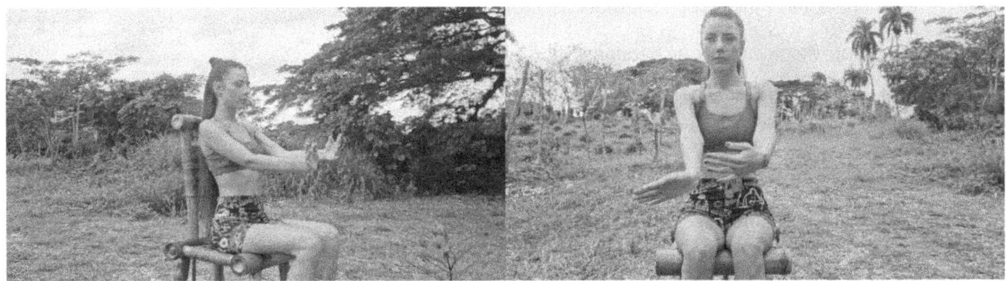

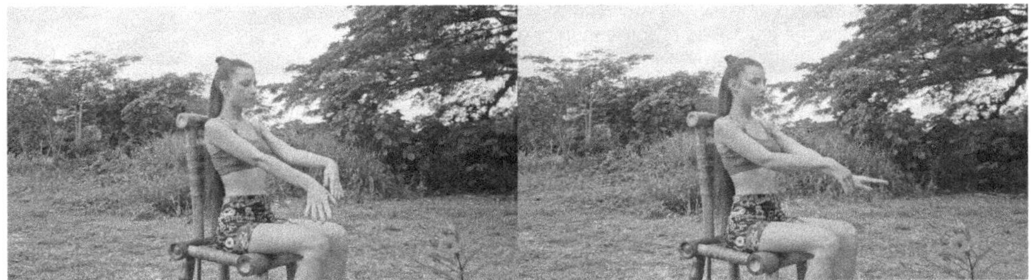

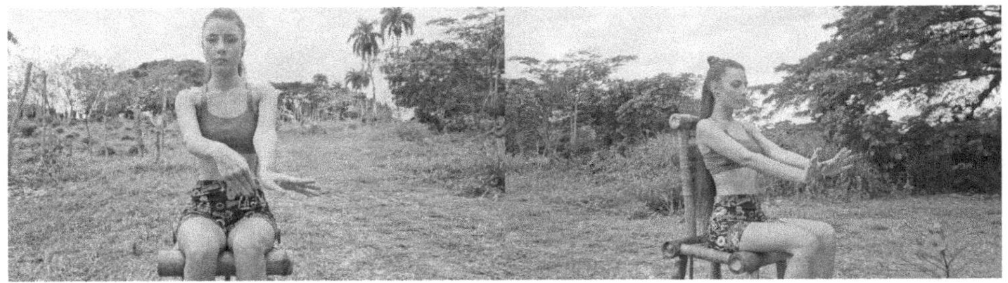

https://youtu.be/B7g44e5XVdA

- Begin in a comfortable seated position with feet flat on the ground.

• Extend your arms forward, palms facing down.

• Gently start making circular motions with your wrists.

• Rotate clockwise for 30 seconds, then switch to counterclockwise.

• Keep the movements small and controlled.

• Feel a gentle stretch in your wrists and forearms.

• If you experience discomfort, reduce the range of motion.

• Continue for 1-2 minutes, then slowly relax your wrists.

• Return your hands to your knees, and take a moment to appreciate the increased mobility in your wrists.

5. Seated Forward Bend

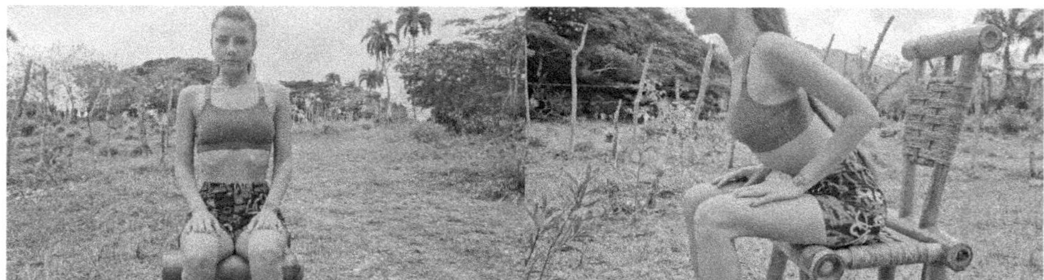

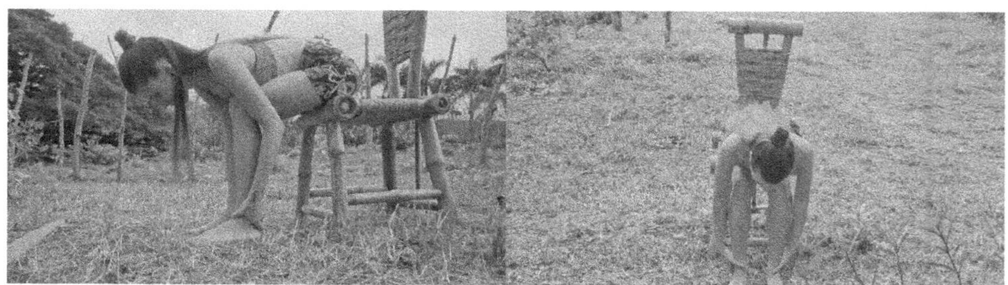

https://youtu.be/iq-wgRWKQoA

• Sit comfortably with your feet flat on the ground, hip-width apart.

• Keep your back straight and your hands resting on your thighs.

• Inhale deeply, lengthening your spine.

• Exhale slowly, hinging at your hips, and lean forward.

• Reach your hands towards your feet without straining.

• Feel a gentle stretch in your lower back and hamstrings.

• Hold the forward bend for 15-30 seconds, breathing steadily.

• Keep your neck relaxed, and let your head hang naturally.

• Inhale as you slowly return to an upright position.

• Take a moment to notice the increased flexibility in your lower back and hamstrings.

6. Ankle Rolls

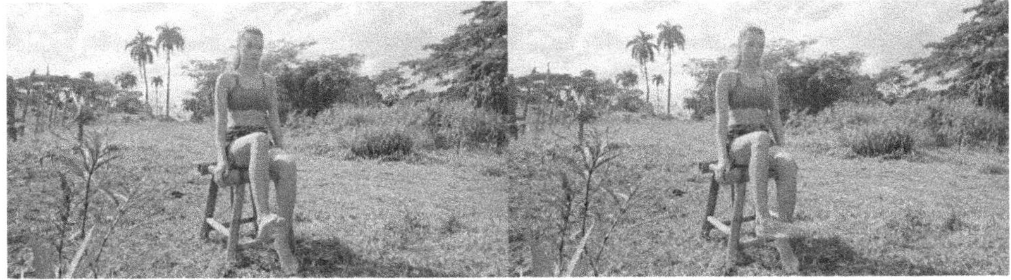

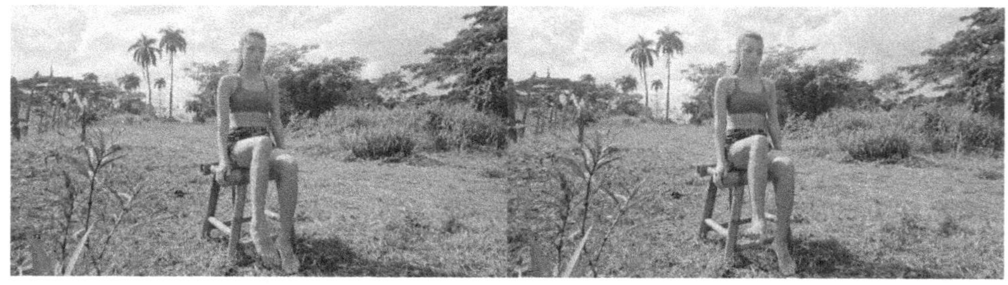

https://youtu.be/pdBis6sIv4c

- Sit comfortably with your feet flat on the ground.
- Lift one foot and gently rotate your ankle clockwise.
- After 30 seconds, switch to counterclockwise rotations.
- Repeat the process with the other foot.
- Perform two sets for each ankle, promoting flexibility.

7. Seated Side Stretch

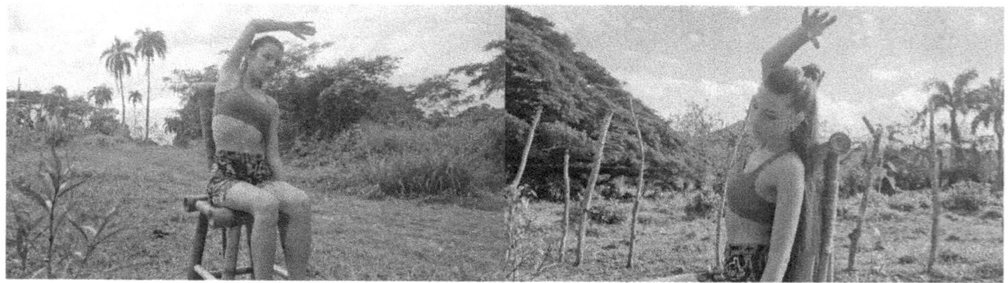

https://youtu.be/8uKTsVGwq3s

- Start in a relaxed seated position with feet flat on the ground.
- Extend your right arm overhead, reaching towards the left.
- Feel a gentle stretch along the right side of your torso.
- Hold for 15-30 seconds, breathing steadily.
- Return to the center and switch to the other side.
- Repeat the stretch on the left side for balance.
- Perform two sets on each side, improving flexibility to reach the sides.

8. Shoulder Shrugs

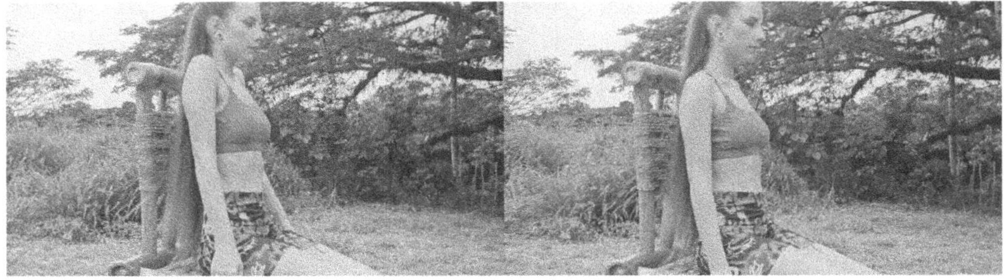

https://youtu.be/94ooQjvrkrg

- Sit comfortably with your feet flat on the ground.
- Lift your shoulders towards your ears.
- Hold for a moment, then release them down.
- Repeat the motion for 1 minute.
- This exercise helps release tension in your shoulders.

9. Seated Twist

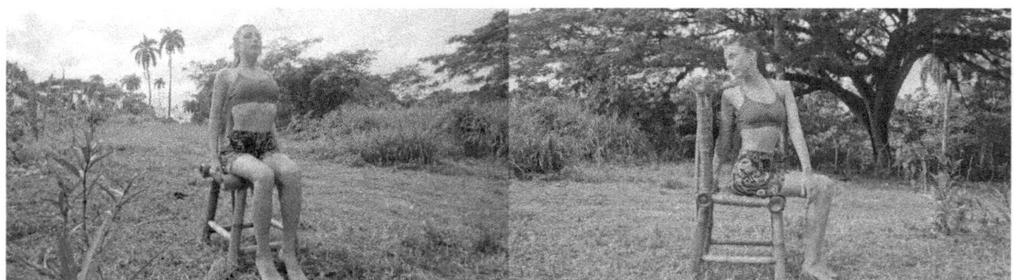

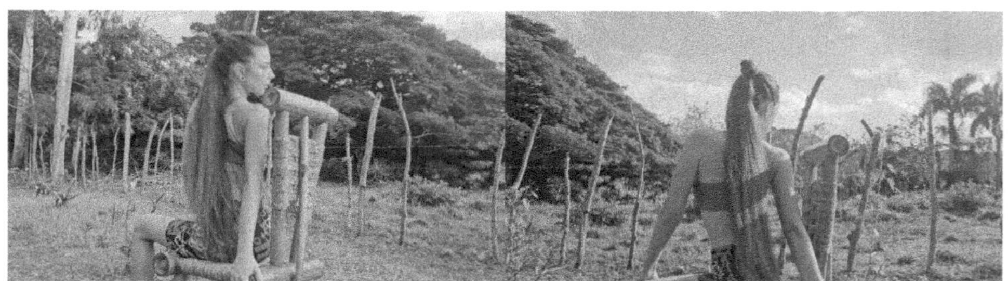

https://youtu.be/27D7DMcG4bQ

- Begin in a relaxed seated position.
- Inhale, lengthen your spine and twist to the right.

- Place your left hand on your right knee and the right hand behind you.
- Hold for 15-30 seconds, breathing deeply.
- Return to the center and repeat on the other side.
- Perform two sets on each side for a gentle spinal twist.

10. Knee Lifts

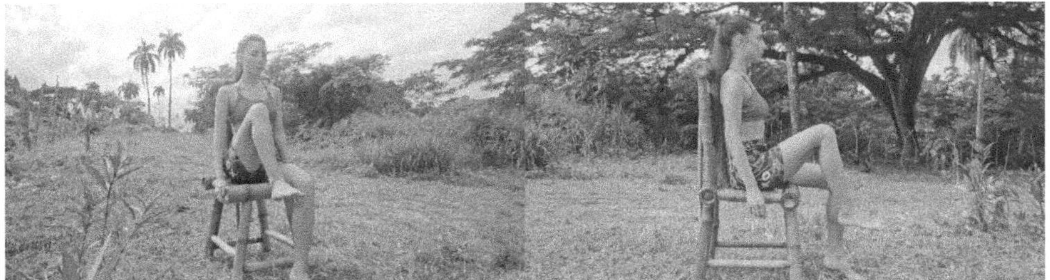

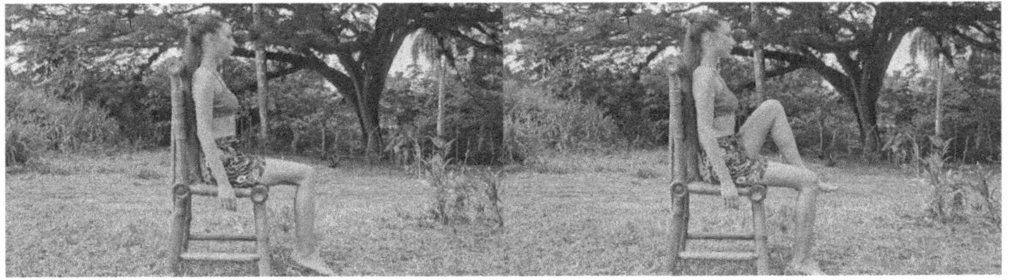

https://youtu.be/2-v6Ly1Dozo

- Sit comfortably with your back straight.
- Lift your right knee towards your chest.
- Hold for a moment, then lower it down.

- Repeat with your left knee.
- Alternate between knees for 1 minute.
- This exercise improves circulation and knee flexibility.

11. Seated Chest Opener

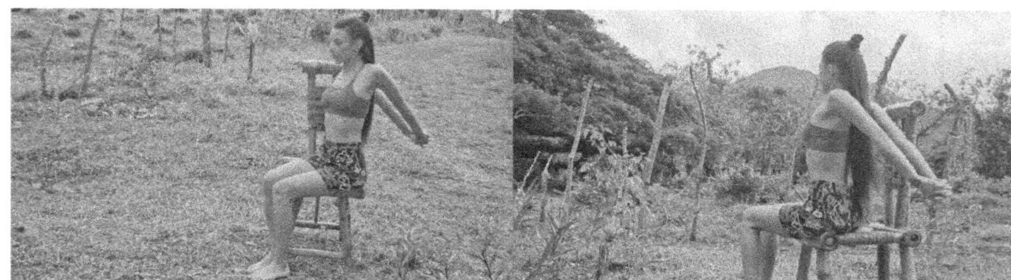

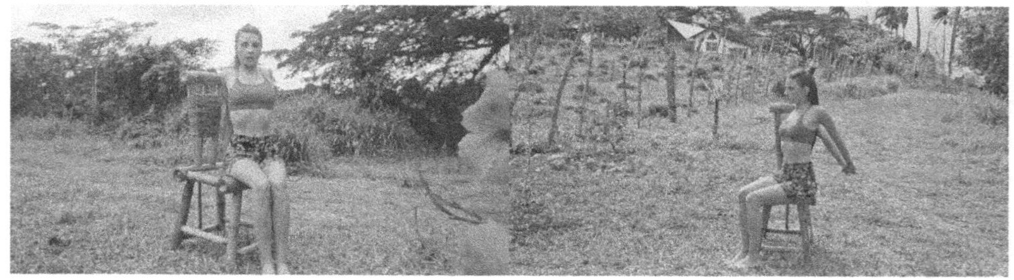

https://youtu.be/N5hDT9SM7vY

- Sit comfortably with your feet flat.
- Clasp your hands behind your back.
- Straighten your arms and lift them slightly.
- Open your chest and hold for 15-30 seconds.

- Release and repeat for two sets.
- This pose promotes chest and shoulder flexibility.

12. Gentle Arm Swings

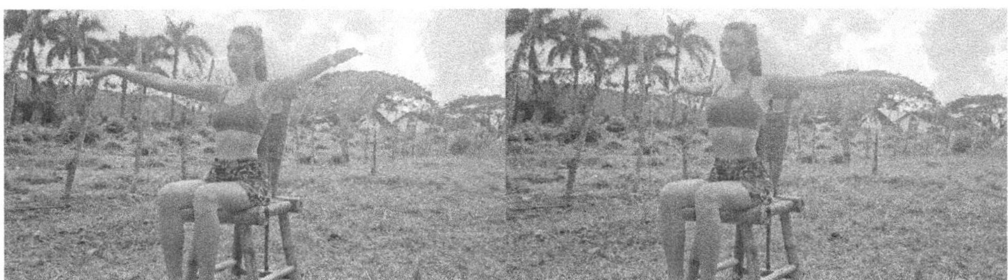

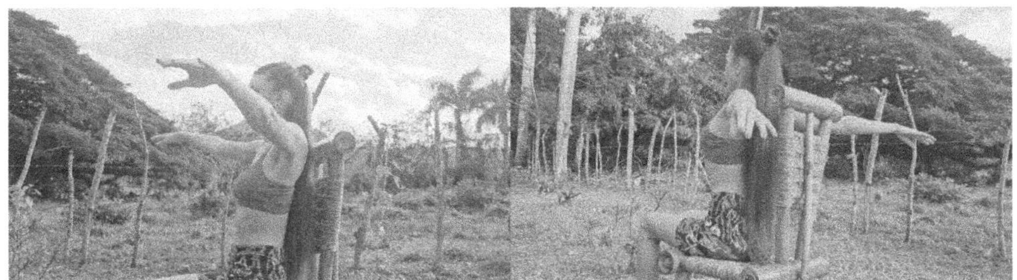

https://youtu.be/_vLhU7uB58o

- Sit comfortably, feet flat on the ground.
- Extend your arms to the sides.
- Swing your arms gently back and forth.
- Maintain a relaxed pace for 1 minute.
- This exercise enhances shoulder mobility.

13. Seated Leg Extension

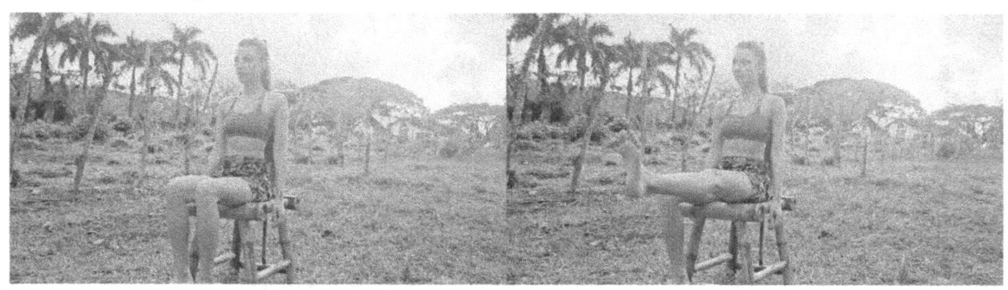

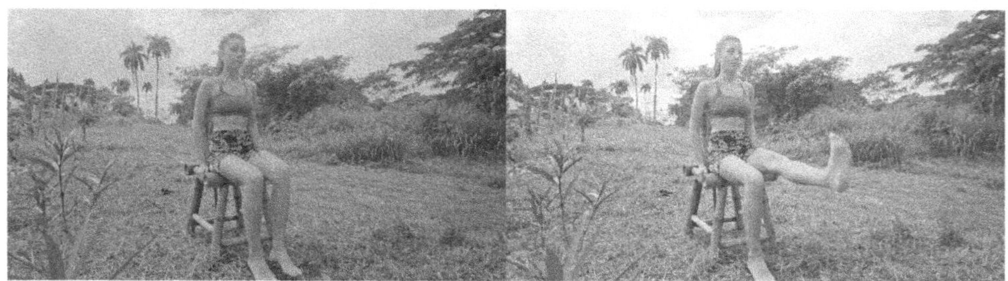

https://youtu.be/hPRfT4xC-rc

- Sit comfortably with your back straight and feet flat.
- Extend one leg forward, keeping it straight.
- Hold for 15-30 seconds, feeling a stretch in your hamstring.
- Return to the starting position and switch legs.
- Repeat for two sets on each leg to enhance leg flexibility.

14. Chest Circles

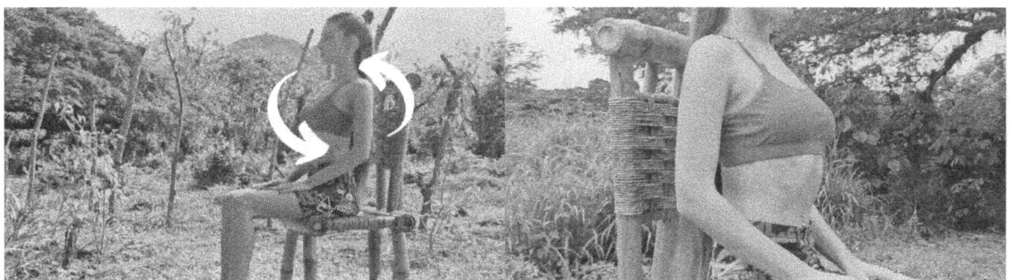

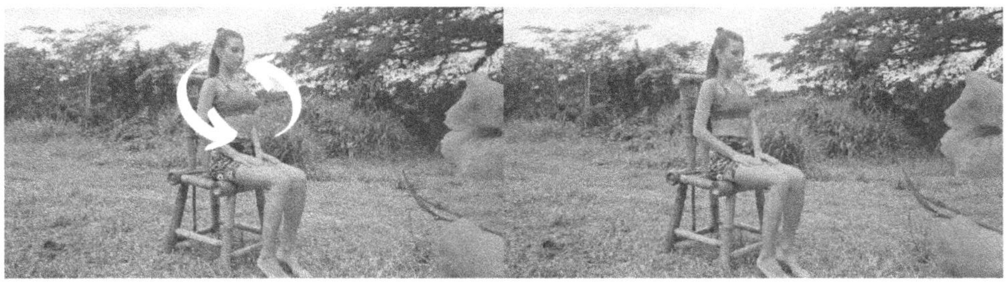

https://youtu.be/lxsOWQg2ozA

- Sit comfortably with your hands on your thighs.
- Circle your chest to the right for 30 seconds.
- Then, circle to the left for another 30 seconds.
- Maintain a smooth and controlled motion.
- This exercise promotes chest and upper back flexibility.

15. Seated Hip Opener

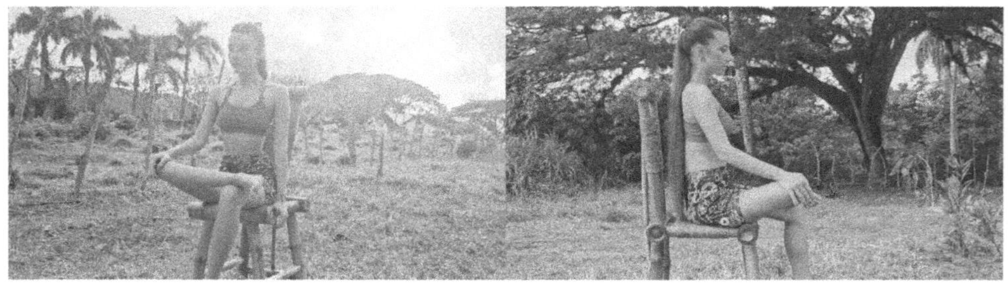

https://youtu.be/yrCENVzwHcE

- Sit with your feet flat and knees bent.
- Place your right ankle on your left knee.
- Gently press down on your right knee.
- Hold for 15-30 seconds, feeling a stretch in your hip.
- Switch legs and repeat for two sets on each side.

16. Seated Rowing Motion

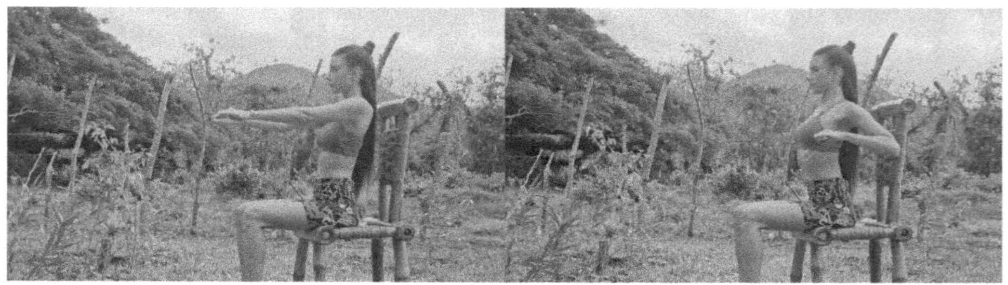

https://youtu.be/FVi3xnriAKo

- Sit comfortably with a straight back.
- Mimic rowing by bringing your arms back and forth.
- Perform the motion for 1 minute, engaging your back muscles.
- This exercise enhances upper back strength and mobility.

17. Seated Knee Hug

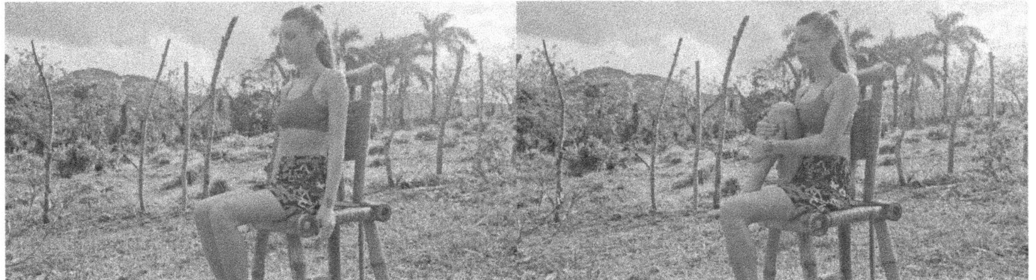

https://youtu.be/WUkuA-ierrk

- Sit comfortably with your back straight.
- Lift your right knee towards your chest.
- Hug it with both hands, holding for 15-30 seconds.
- Switch to the left knee and repeat for two sets.

• This pose stretches your lower back and hip flexors.

18. Finger Stretch

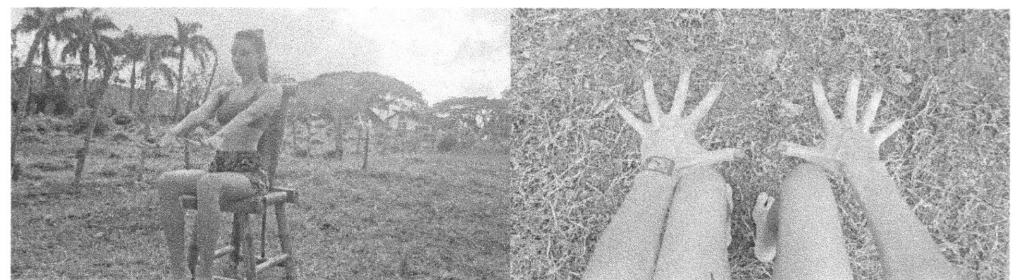

https://youtu.be/3piOTh6eozU

• Sit comfortably with your back straight and hands resting on your thighs.

• Extend your fingers wide, spreading them apart.

• Hold the stretch for 10-15 seconds, feeling the tension in your fingers.

• Relax and then repeat the stretch for two sets.

• This exercise helps improve finger flexibility and reduces stiffness.

19. Seated Side-to-Side Movement

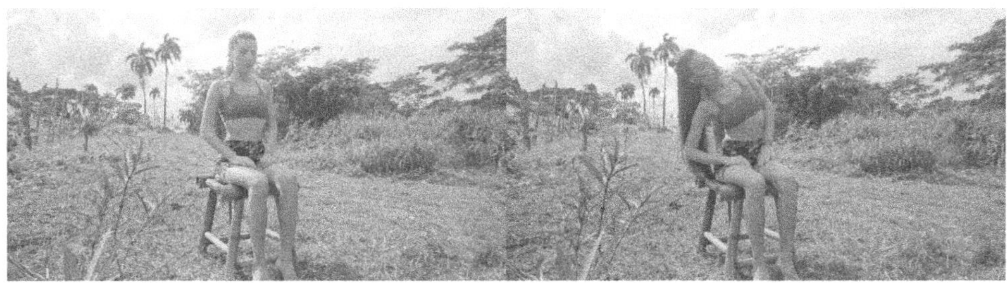

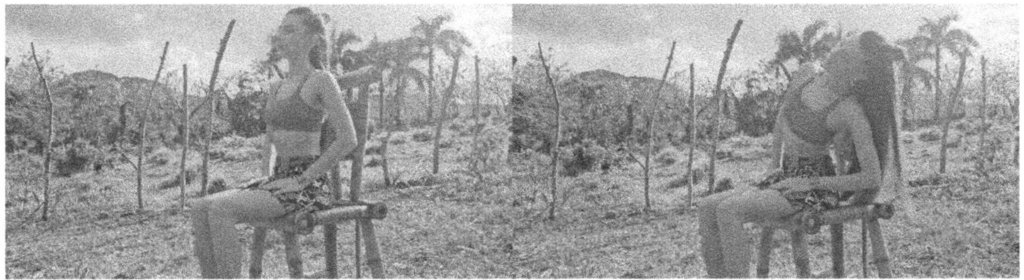

https://youtu.be/dUHr3oRoEEs

- Begin in a relaxed seated position with your feet flat on the ground.
- Gently sway your upper body to the right side, feeling a stretch along your left side.
- Hold for 15-30 seconds, breathing naturally.
- Return to the center and repeat the movement to the left side.
- Perform two sets on each side, promoting lateral flexibility.

20. Toe Taps

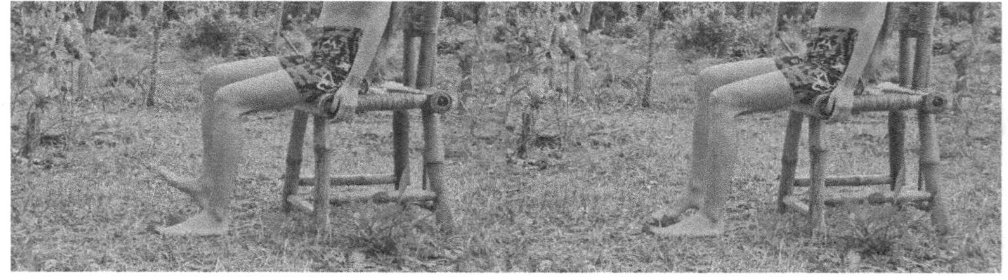

https://youtu.be/2Pt6quHAxqc

- Sit with your back straight and feet flat on the ground.
- Lift your right foot, tapping your toes on the ground.
- Alternate between feet in a rhythmic motion.
- Continue for 1 minute, engaging your leg muscles.
- This exercise improves circulation and warms up your legs.

21. Seated Spinal Flex

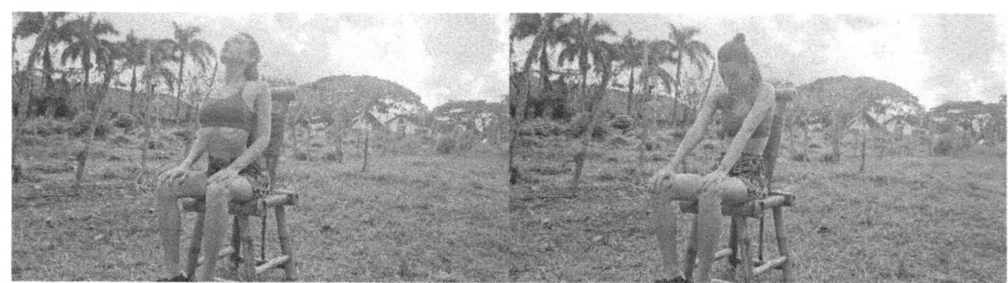

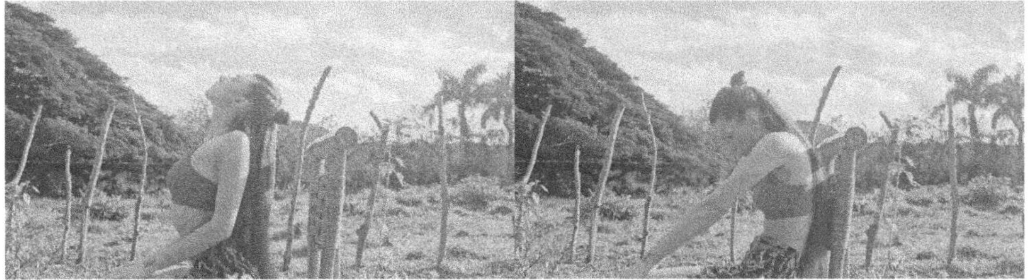

https://youtu.be/Uq4UxWhMFRM

- Sit comfortably with your hands on your knees.
- Inhale, arching your back and lifting your chest.
- Exhale, rounding your back and tucking your chin.
- Repeat this flexing motion for 1-2 minutes.
- Enhances flexibility and mobility in your spine.

22. Pelvic Tilts

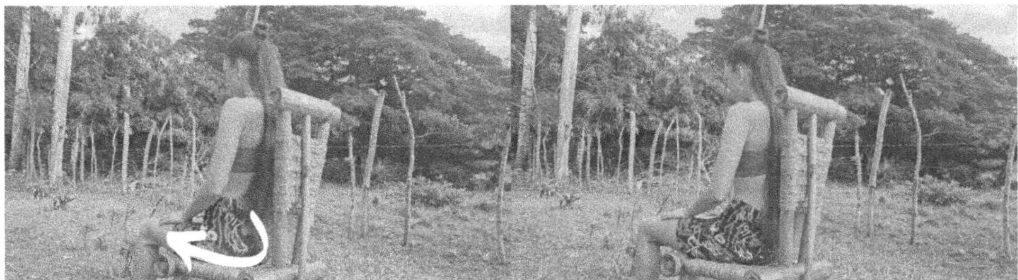

https://youtu.be/Z36yYKeLeR8

- Sit with your feet flat and your hands on your thighs.
- Tilt your pelvis forward, arching your lower back.
- Then, tilt it backward, rounding your lower back.
- Repeat for 1 minute, coordinating with your breath.
- Strengthens and loosens your pelvic muscles.

23. Seated Calf Stretch

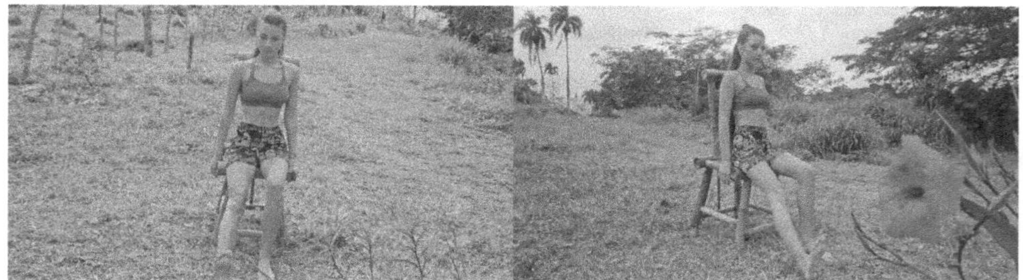

https://youtu.be/oL4qRuPAwG8

- Sit with your feet flat on the ground.
- Extend one leg forward, flexing your foot.
- Hold for 15-30 seconds, feeling the stretch in your calf.

- Switch legs and repeat for two sets on each side.
- This stretch targets your calf muscles effectively.

24. Deep Breathing Exercise

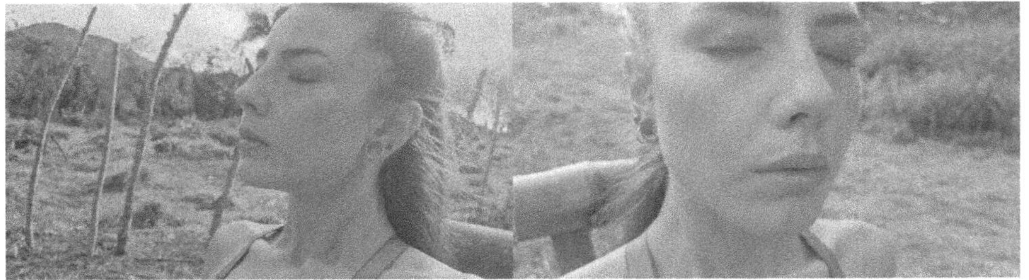

https://youtu.be/ZWz7YziB_UA

- Sit comfortably, close your eyes, and relax your shoulders.
- Inhale deeply through your nose for a count of four.
- Exhale slowly through your mouth for a count of six.
- Repeat this deep breathing pattern for 2 minutes.
- A calming exercise to promote relaxation and focus.

25. Seated Figure 8 Arm Movement

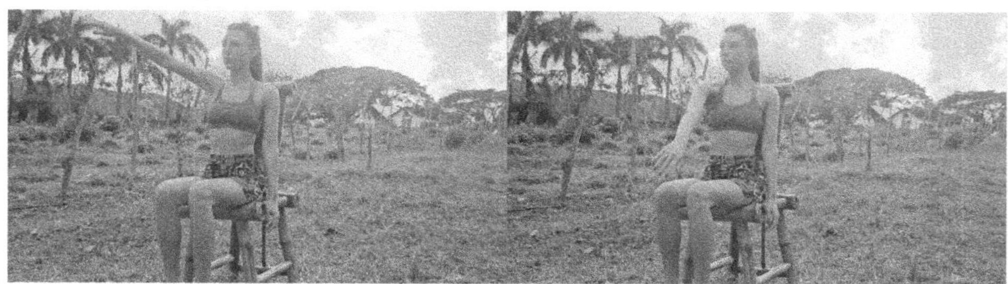

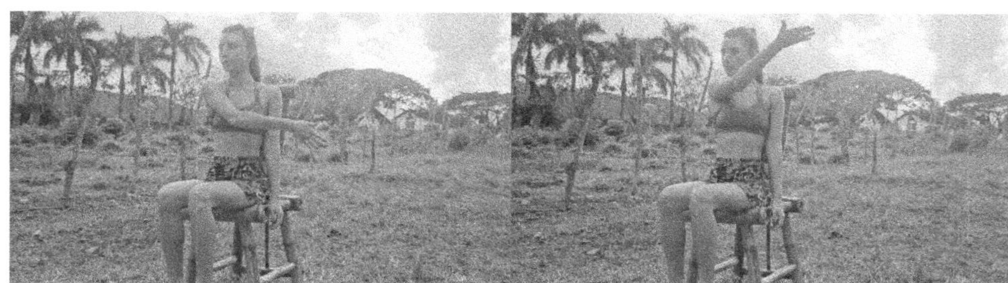

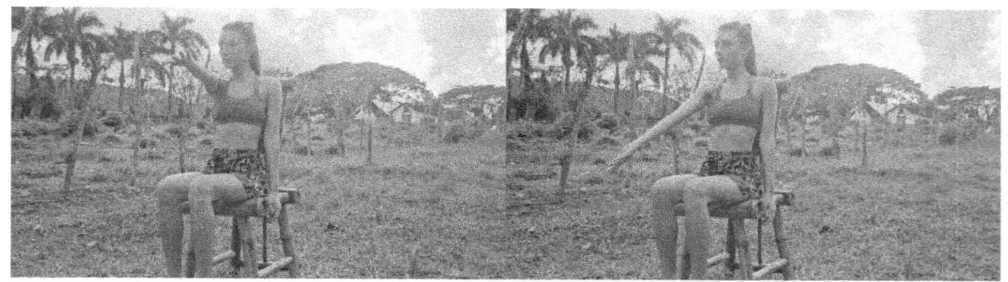

https://youtu.be/OFDRRYjTkzo

- Sit with your feet flat on the ground and back straight.
- Lift your right arm, tracing a figure-eight motion in the air.

- Repeat with your left arm.
- Continue for 1-2 minutes, promoting shoulder mobility.
- This exercise enhances arm flexibility and coordination.

Variations and Modifications for Different Abilities

Yoga poses are incredibly adaptable, and modifications can be implemented to cater to your capacities. Listen to your body, prioritize comfort, and adjust as needed. For those with limited mobility or flexibility, consider the following general guidance to modify poses: (Schettler, 2021)

Seated Mountain Pose

Standard Pose: Sit at the front of the chair with feet flat on the ground.

Modification: Place a cushion or folded blanket under your hips for added support for those with limited flexibility. Gradually increase elevation as you become more comfortable.

Neck Tilts and Turns

Standard Pose: Tilt and turn your head slowly, feeling gentle stretches.

Modification: If sitting upright is challenging, perform these movements while comfortably reclining in the chair. Adjust the range of motion to ensure a pain-free experience.

Seated Leg Extension

Standard Pose: Extend one leg forward while keeping the other foot flat on the ground.

Modification: If lifting your leg is challenging, focus on extending it just slightly or use a resistance band around the foot for assistance. Gradually increase the range of motion over time.

Incorporate these modifications as needed, and always prioritize safety and comfort. Remember that the essence of yoga lies in adapting the practice to suit your unique needs, ensuring a positive and fulfilling experience.

Personalized Poses for Specific Health Conditions

Health Conditions Chair Yoga Can Help With

Chair yoga offers a versatile and accessible way to address various health conditions. Tailoring poses and adjusting them to specific needs can provide targeted benefits for individuals with health challenges. Below are chair yoga poses categorized based on the health conditions they can help alleviate: (flowithmeie, 2020)

Arthritis

Wrist Circles: Wrist circles are particularly beneficial for individuals with arthritis in the hands. The gentle circular motions help enhance wrist flexibility without causing strain. This promotes joint mobility and can alleviate stiffness commonly associated with hand arthritis.

Seated Knee Hug: Seated knee hugs provide a targeted solution for arthritis affecting the lower body. By lifting the knees towards the chest, this pose promotes joint mobility and helps individuals with arthritis in the hips or knees find relief. The gentle action improves flexibility without putting undue stress on the joints.

Seated Chest Opener: Arthritis-related discomfort in the upper body, particularly in the chest and shoulders, can be relieved through the seated chest opener. This pose involves gentle stretches that release stiffness, providing comfort for individuals with arthritis in the upper extremities.

Back Pain

Seated Forward Bend: The seated forward bend is a valuable pose for individuals struggling with chronic back pain. By gently stretching the lower back and hamstrings, this pose helps alleviate tension and promotes flexibility. It is an accessible yet effective way to address discomfort associated with back pain.

Seated Spinal Flex: Individuals dealing with back pain can benefit from the seated spinal flex. This pose involves gentle flexing motions that improve spinal flexibility. By incorporating this into a routine, individuals can ease tension in the back, ensuring greater comfort and mobility.

Seated Leg Extension (Modified): Tailored for those with back pain, the modified seated leg extension allows a gradual extension of the legs with added support. This pose provides the benefits of leg extension without straining the lower back, offering relief to individuals managing back pain.

Poses for Osteoporosis

Seated Knee Hug: Seated knee hugs are gentle yet effective for individuals with osteoporosis. This pose promotes flexibility and joint mobility without excessive stress on the bones. The controlled movement aids in enhancing overall lower body strength.

Seated Chest Opener: Osteoporosis often affects the spine and chest area. The seated chest opener provides a gentle stretch that helps maintain flexibility in the chest and upper back. This can result in improved posture and reduced strain on the spine.

Seated Leg Extension (Modified): The modified seated leg extension offers a safe way to work on leg strength for individuals with osteoporosis. With added support, the controlled extension ensures that the exercise is beneficial without putting undue pressure on vulnerable areas.

Poses for Anxiety and Stress

Deep Breathing Exercise: Deep breathing exercises are paramount for managing anxiety and stress. This seated exercise involves slow, intentional inhalations through the nose and extended exhalations through the mouth, promoting relaxation and calming the nervous system.

Seated Chest Opener: Anxiety and stress often manifest as tension in the chest and shoulders. The seated chest opener helps release this tension, allowing individuals to experience a sense of openness and ease in the upper body.

Seated Forward Bend: The seated forward bend is an excellent pose for relieving stress. As individuals fold forward, the pose encourages a sense of surrender and relaxation, relieving tension in the back and promoting mental calmness.

Poses for Circulation Issues

Toe Taps: Toe taps are a simple yet effective way to promote circulation in the lower extremities. The rhythmic movement stimulates blood flow to the legs, benefiting individuals with circulation issues.

Seated Figure 8 Arm Movement: The seated figure 8 arm movement is an excellent choice for improved circulation in the arms and shoulders. The continuous motion enhances blood flow, providing a gentle workout for the upper body.

Knee Lifts (Modified): Modified knee lifts, done while seated, enhance overall circulation. This controlled movement engages the leg muscles, facilitating blood flow without excessive strain on the cardiovascular system.

Adding these personalized chair yoga poses into a routine can offer targeted benefits for individuals managing osteoporosis, anxiety and stress, and circulation issues. Always consult a healthcare provider, especially when dealing with specific health conditions.

Incorporating Personalized Poses

Tailoring chair yoga poses to address specific health conditions involves selecting exercises that target the affected areas or offer relief. Here's how you can customize your chair yoga practice:

Identify the Target Area: For arthritis, focus on poses that promote flexibility in the affected joints, such as gentle leg and wrist movements. For back pain, emphasize exercises that strengthen the core and promote spinal flexibility.

Modify Intensity: Adjust the intensity of poses based on individual comfort levels. For those with arthritis, gentler and more controlled movements are advisable. Individuals with back pain may benefit from gradually increasing the range of motion as they become more comfortable.

Consultation with a Professional: All the chair yoga practices incorporated in this book are safe for seniors. If you need further guidance on your underlying medical conditions, you must consult your doctor and safely incorporate these chair yoga poses.

Personalizing chair yoga poses for specific health conditions empowers individuals to address their unique needs, creating a sense of optimal health and comfort.

* * *

Daily Planner for a 10-Minute Chair Yoga Routine

Warm-Up (2 minutes):	**Seated Neck Tilts and Turns (30 seconds):** Gently begin with seated neck tilts and turns to loosen up neck muscles and improve flexibility. **Wrist Circles (30 seconds):** Engage in wrist circles to warm up the wrists and enhance mobility, which is especially beneficial for those with arthritis. **Seated Chest Opener (1 minute):** Open up the chest to release tension and enhance breathing, beneficial for stress relief.
Main Poses (6 minutes):	**Seated Mountain Pose (1 minute):** Establish a solid foundation, promoting stability and improved posture. Seated Chest Opener (1 minute): Open up the chest to release tension and enhance breathing, which is beneficial for stress relief. **Seated Forward Bend (1 minute):** Stretch the lower back and hamstrings, resulting in better flexibility and relaxation. **Seated Leg Extension (1 minute):** Promote leg strength and flexibility with controlled leg extensions, adaptable for various abilities. **Deep Breathing Exercise (1 minute):** Engage in deep breathing to calm the mind and promote relaxation, which is necessary for overall harmony. **Seated Shoulder Shrugs (1 minute):** Elevate and lower your shoulders to release tension in the upper back and shoulders.
Cool Down (2 minutes):	**Seated Spinal Flex (30 seconds):** Cool down with seated spinal flex to ease tension in the back and enhance spinal flexibility. **Seated Figure 8 Arm Movement (30 seconds):** Wind down with gentle arm movements, promoting circulation and relaxation. **Seated Knee Hug (1 minute):** Finish with a seated knee hug to relax the lower back and hips, providing a soothing end to the routine.

Summary of the daily planner:

This 10-minute chair yoga routine offers a well-rounded experience, incorporating a brief warm-up, various seated poses targeting different areas, and a calming cool-down.

Weekly Goal Setting and Progress Tracking

Setting fitness goals and tracking progress is crucial to maintaining a successful chair yoga routine. Here are simple steps to set realistic goals and monitor your progress:

Define Clear and Achievable Goals: Identify specific, measurable, and realistic goals. For example, aim to increase the duration of chair yoga sessions or improve flexibility in targeted areas.

Create a Weekly Plan: Establish a weekly plan by allocating specific days and times for chair yoga. Consistency is key, so choose a schedule that aligns with daily routines.

Start with Realistic Targets: For beginners, start with achievable targets. This could involve gradually increasing the number of poses, extending the duration of sessions, or trying new poses that challenge but are not overwhelming.

Use a Chair Yoga Journal: Maintain a chair yoga journal to record goals, daily practices, and observations. This provides a tangible record of progress and allows for reflection on achievements.

Monitor Flexibility and Comfort: Keep track of improvements in flexibility and overall comfort during poses. Note any changes in range of motion or reduced discomfort, which are indicators of progress.

Set Mindfulness Goals: Consider incorporating mindfulness goals, such as focusing on breath awareness or reducing stress levels during sessions. These objectives contribute to both mental and physical health.

Gradual Intensity Increase: As comfort levels improve, the intensity of chair yoga poses gradually increases. This might involve holding poses longer or exploring more advanced variations.

Celebrate Small Wins: Acknowledge and celebrate small victories. Whether it's achieving a new pose or completing a session without discomfort, these milestones are significant indicators of progress.

Periodic Assessments: Conduct regular assessments to evaluate overall improvement. Assessments may include revisiting initial goals, comparing flexibility levels, and adjusting the routine.

Adjust and Adapt: Adjust goals based on individual needs and circumstances. Adapt the routine to accommodate fitness level changes or address new focus areas.

Final Words

As we conclude this chapter on establishing a fulfilling chair yoga routine, it's wise to recall the wise words of Gandhi: "It is health that is real wealth and not pieces of gold and silver." In alignment with this philosophy, we've explored the foundations of chair yoga, advancing into beginner poses with a focus on simplicity, adaptability, and overall harmony.

Key Takeaways

Accessible Wellness: Chair yoga provides an accessible avenue for individuals of all abilities to embark on a wellness journey. Its simplicity and adaptability make it a valuable practice for enhancing physical and mental health.

Daily Routine Blueprint: The provided daily planner empowers readers to integrate chair yoga seamlessly into their lives, offering a structured routine that accommodates warm-up, main poses, and cool-down exercises in just 10 minutes.

As we move forward, Chapter 5 awaits, offering a progression to "Step #5: Mastering Intermediate Poses." Building upon the knowledge gained, we will explore new poses that challenge and elevate the practice. Get ready to take the next step in your chair yoga journey, unlocking a deeper level of flexibility, strength, and mindfulness.

* * *

TAKE A MOMENT TO PLEASE LEAVE A REVIEW

Hey, awesome readers!
Dived into "The Ultimate Illustrated Guide to Chair Yoga for Seniors Over 60" and loved it? Think how your review could help someone else start their own chair yoga adventure. Sharing your thoughts isn't just feedback; it's a beacon for others contemplating this journey, showing them the benefits and joys of chair yoga.

We'd love for you to share your experience. It could be a quick shout-out or a few sincere words – your genuine review will light the way for others. Just head to amzn.to/4aTg2n5 or scan the QR Code to leave your review.

USA UK CAN

Your insights have the potential to inspire change, guiding others to a happier, healthier life. Plus, you'll join a community championing wellness and togetherness.
Let's create ripples of positivity. Your review isn't just feedback; it's an invitation to wellness and connection. Share the chair yoga love, one review at a time.

Step #5: Mastering Intermediate Poses

"Exercise to stimulate, not to annihilate. The world wasn't formed in a day, and neither were we. Set small goals and build upon them." —Lee Haney.

Welcome to Chapter 5—Mastering Intermediate Poses. In this chapter, we'll take a focused approach, encouraging you to elevate your practice by introducing a set of intermediate poses. Keep reading and find your way to mastering these poses and gaining guidance for safe and effective progression. As Lee Haney said, progress is a gradual process, and the same applies to your yoga practice. By setting small goals and building upon them, you're on the path to mastering the intricacies of chair yoga.

In the following pages, we will discuss each pose with clear, step-by-step instructions, allowing you to advance your practice comfortably.

25 Intermediate Chair Yoga Poses for Increased Strength and Flexibility

This section will explore a curated collection of intermediate chair yoga poses designed to intensify your practice, gradually bringing increased strength and flexibility to work. Each pose is chosen to provide a unique challenge while considering the supportive nature of chair yoga. Now, let's begin with the first pose:

1. Seated Peaceful Warrior Pose

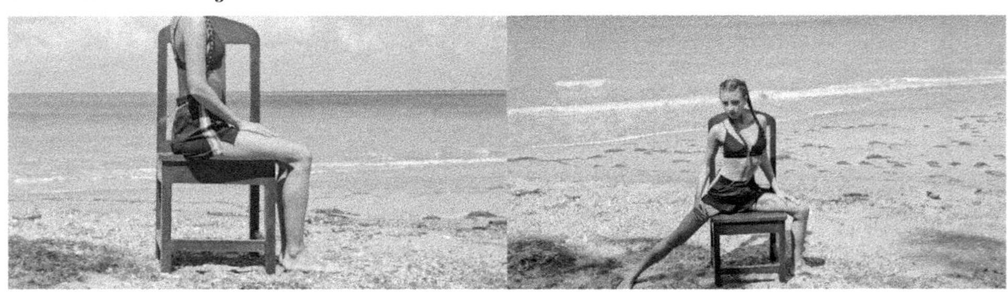

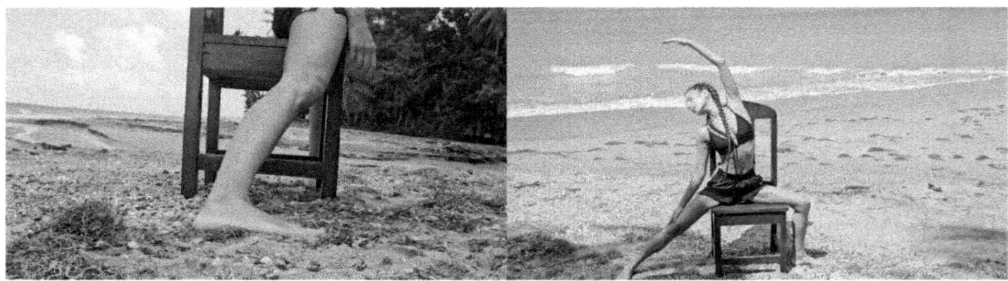

https://youtu.be/e43NsCdrJSk

- Sit on your chair with your left side facing the backrest of the chair, and with your feet planted.
- Inhale, lengthen the spine, and engage the core.
- Exhale, extend the right leg backwards flexing the foot.
- Inhale, raise the left arm overhead, creating a gentle side stretch.
- Hold and breathe, feeling engagement in the core.
- Return to the starting position and repeat on the other side.

Tip: Maintain smooth, controlled movements and a comfortable stretch.

2. Dynamic Chair Squats

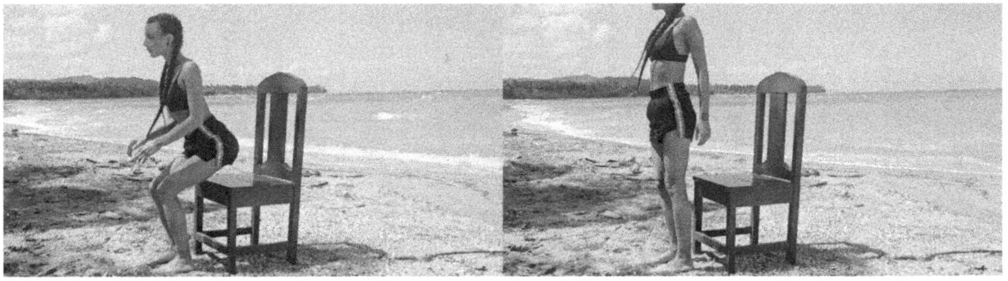

https://youtu.be/n7vY1KM8evw

- Sit comfortably, feet hip-width apart.
- Inhale, stand up, extending hips and knees.
- Exhale, slowly lower back into a seated position.
- Repeat for 10-15 reps, maintaining a controlled pace.
- Focus on engaging the quadriceps and glutes.

Tip: Keep chest lifted, and ensure knees align with ankles during squats.

3. Seated Eagle Arms

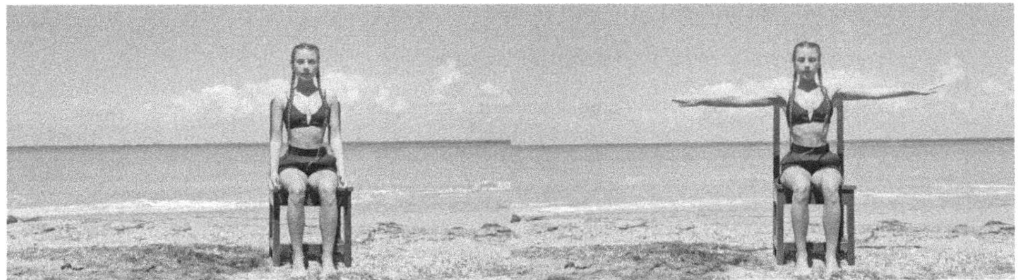

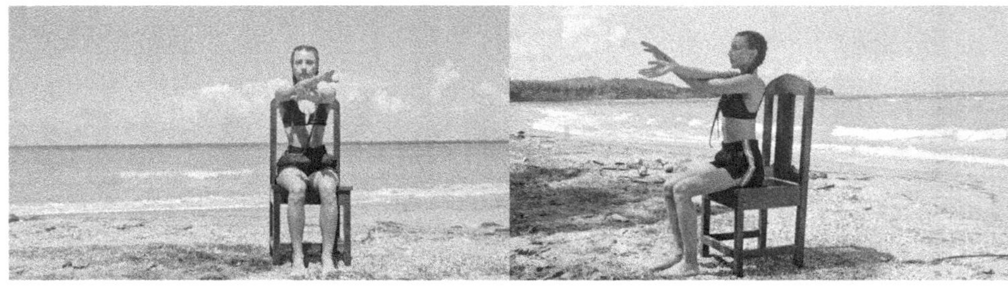

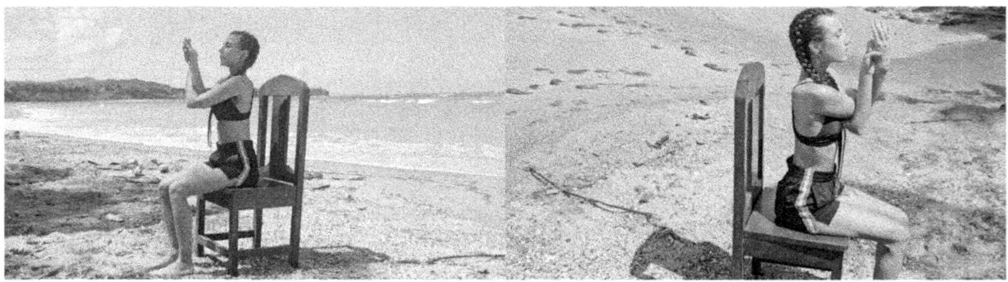

https://youtu.be/zRLPrFQH5qU

- Sit tall, feet flat on the floor.
- Inhale, extend arms to the sides.
- Exhale, cross right arm over left, palms together.
- Lift elbows slightly, feeling a stretch between shoulder blades.
- Hold for several breaths, then switch arm position.

Tip: If palms don't touch, hold onto shoulders with hands.

4. Hip Flexor Stretch

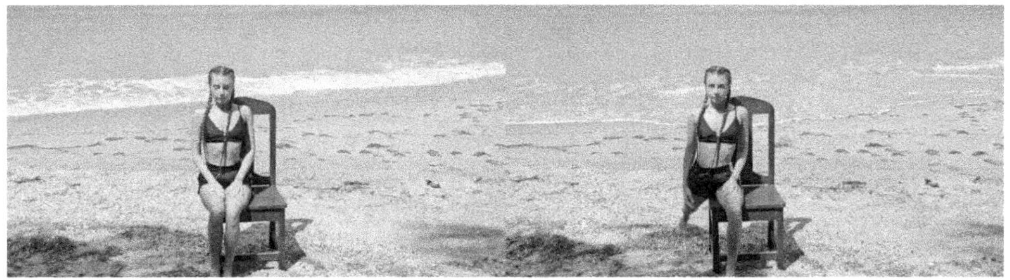

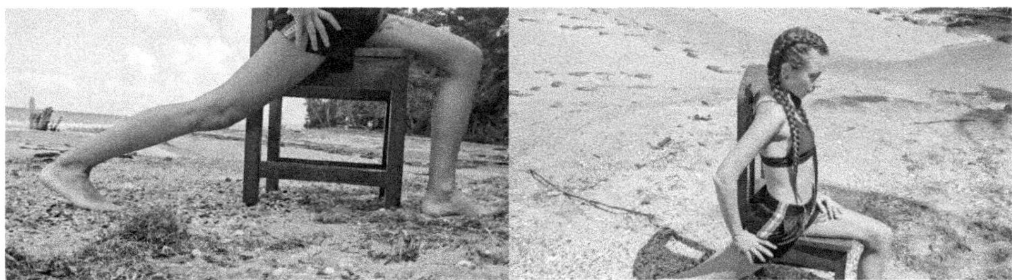

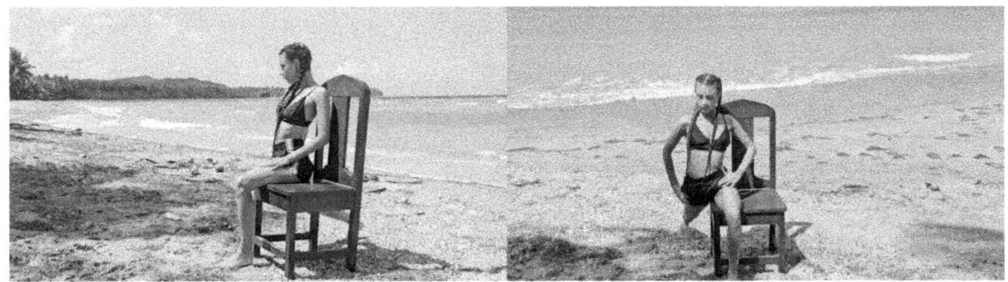

https://youtu.be/kCfJAirlA2w

- Sit on the right side of the chair with feet flat.
- Extend right leg straight back, flexing your foot on the floor.

• Press the right hip forward, feeling a stretch in the front of the hip.

• Hold for 20-30 seconds, breathing deeply.

• Switch sides and repeat the stretch with the left leg.

Tip: Keep the back straight, avoid arching, and focus on the stretch in the hip flexors.

5. Chair High Lunge

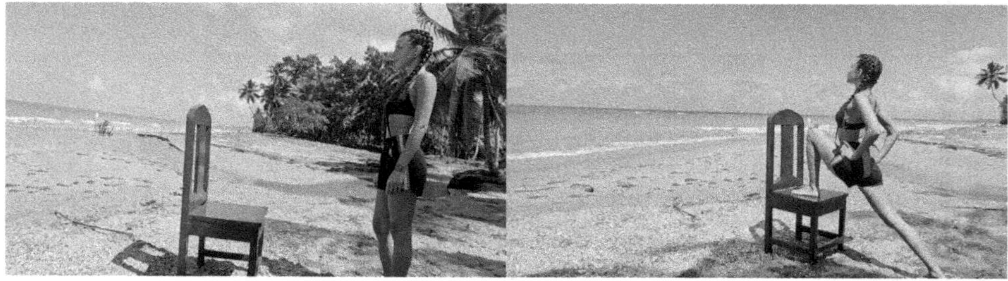

https://youtu.be/YHoZlYZZnGI

• Stand facing the chair, and make a step backward.

• Inhale, lift the left foot off the ground, and place it on the chair, keeping the right foot planted on the ground.

• Keep the chest lifted and engage the core.

• Hold for a few breaths, feeling the stretch in the left hip.

• Return to the starting position and repeat on the other side.

Tip: Focus on stability and balance, maintaining a tall spine throughout.

6. Leg Cross Stretch

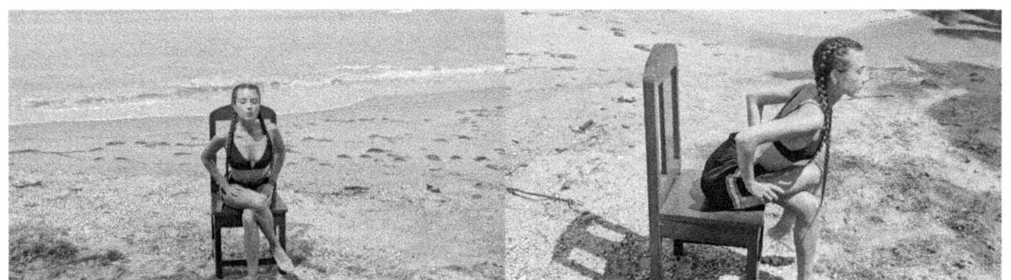

https://youtu.be/cguB9oa8G1s

• Sit comfortably, cross the right leg over the left, placing the left foot on the floor.

• Inhale, lengthen the spine, and exhale, gently hinging forward from the hips.

• Feel the stretch in the outer hip of the crossed leg.

• Hold for 20-30 seconds, then switch the leg position and repeat.

Tip: Keep the back straight and hinge from the hips for a targeted stretch.

7. Seated Tree Pose

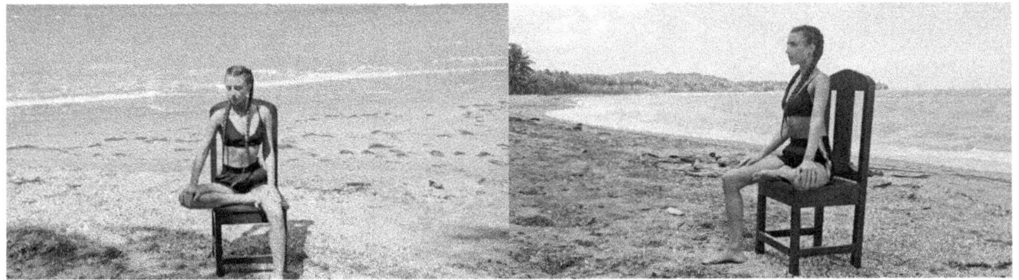

https://youtu.be/bWClXYvXJPY

• Sit tall, spine straight, with feet flat on the floor.

• Lift the right foot, placing it on the inner left thigh.

• Press the right knee down, opening the hip.

• Hold for several breaths, then switch sides.

Tip: Find a focal point to aid balance, and keep the foot on the inner thigh or calf.

8. Tricep Dips

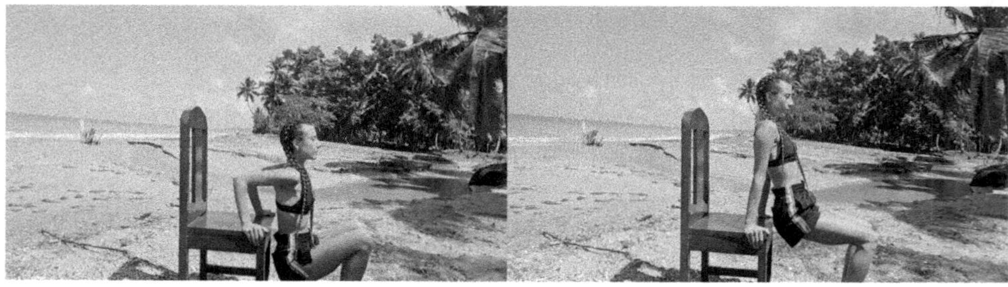

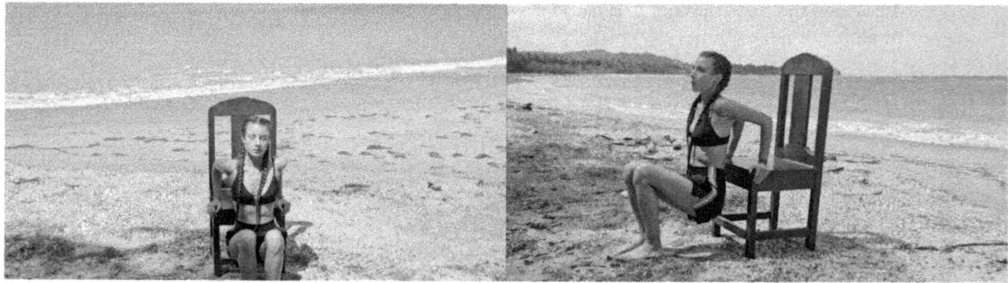

https://youtu.be/2uEUgKiDX7A

- Sit at the edge of the chair, gripping the sides with your hands.
- Slide off the chair, lowering the body with bent elbows.
- Inhale to lower, exhale to push back up.
- Repeat for 10-15 reps, engaging the triceps and core.

Tip: Ensure the elbows point backwards and close to the chair for effective dips.

9. Seated Pigeon Pose

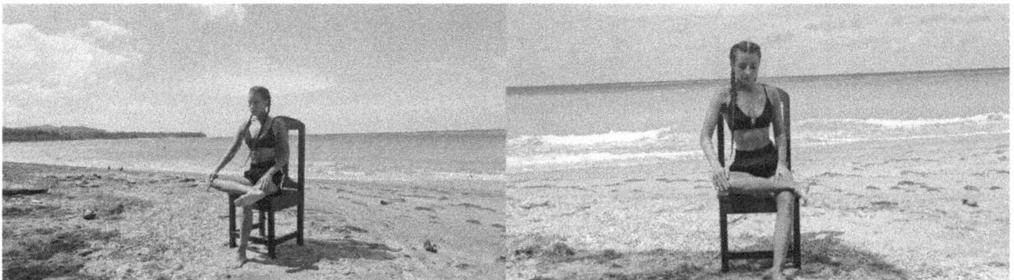

https://youtu.be/TR17TRlao5A

- Sit tall on the chair with both feet flat on the floor (or ground).
- Lift the right leg and place the ankle on the left knee.

• Flex the right foot and gently press the right knee towards the floor/ground.

• Hold for 20-30 seconds, feeling a stretch in the right hip.

• Switch sides and repeat.

Tip: Keep the spine straight and engage the core for a deep hip stretch.

10. Standing Forward Bend

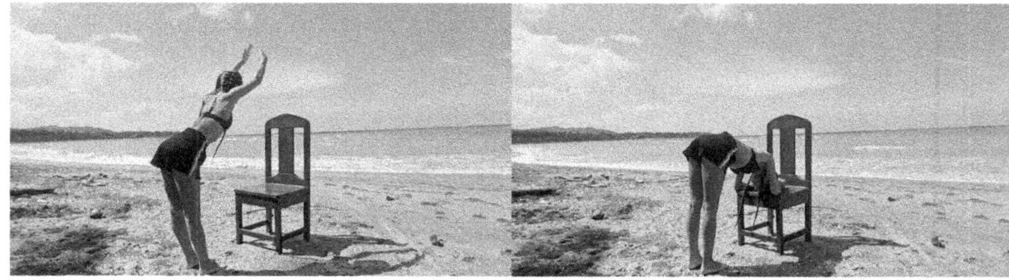

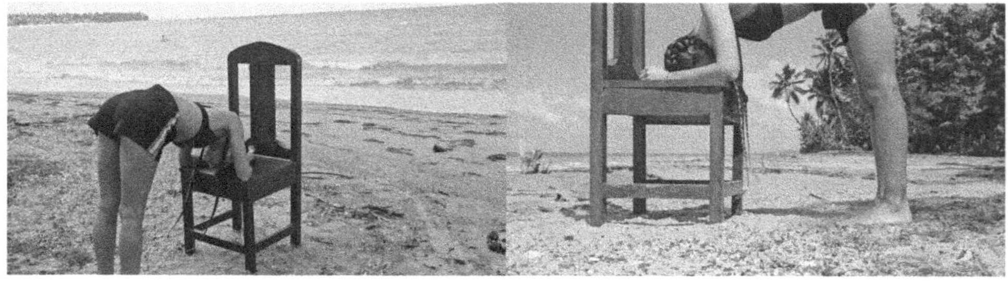

https://youtu.be/mbH7iTSfCug

• Stand facing the chair, feet hip-width apart.

• Inhale, lift the arms overhead.

• Exhale, hinge at the hips, reaching for the chair for support.

• Allow the head and neck to relax.

• Hold for 20-30 seconds, feeling the stretch in the hamstrings and lower back.

Tip: Maintain a slight bend in the knees and focus on lengthening the spine.

11. Chair Side Plank

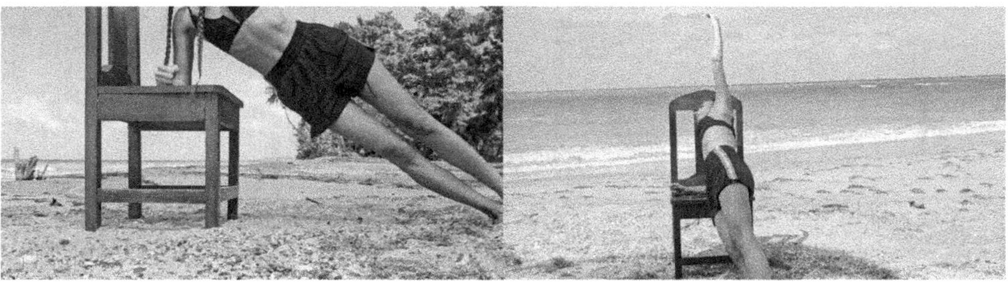

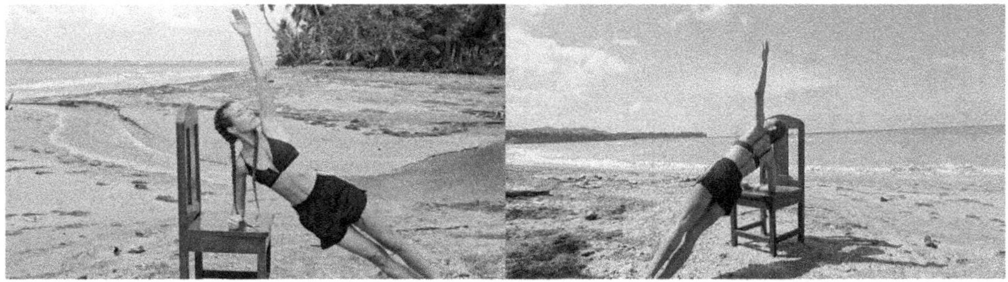

https://youtu.be/5J6UqUfToxo

• Get into a side plank position, with your right elbow on the chair and your feet stacked on the floor.

• Lift the hips, bringing the weight onto the right hand.

• Extend the left arm overhead, creating a straight line from the fingertips to the hips.

• Hold for 15-20 seconds, engaging the core.

• Return to the seated position and switch sides.

Tip: Ensure a strong base and engage the obliques for stability.

12. Hamstring Stretch

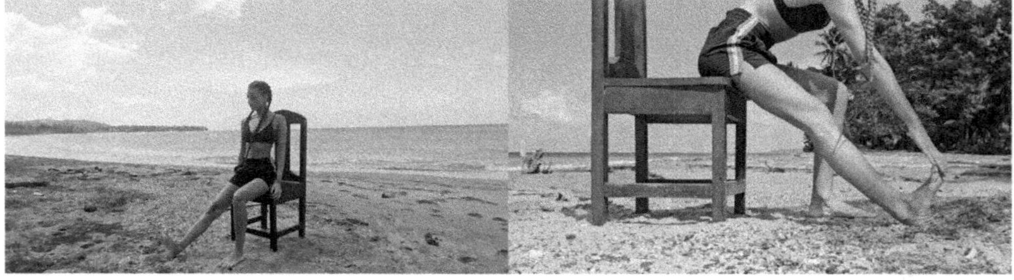

https://youtu.be/JNTIAsMgBi4

• Sit at the edge of the chair with one leg extended.

• Inhale, lengthen the spine, exhale, and hinge at the hips.

• lean forward, reaching for the toes or shins, keeping the back straight.

• Hold for 20-30 seconds, feeling the stretch in the hamstrings.

• Repeat the exercise switching the legs

Tip: Focus on the stretch in the back of the thighs and avoid rounding the back.

13. Seated Sun Salutation

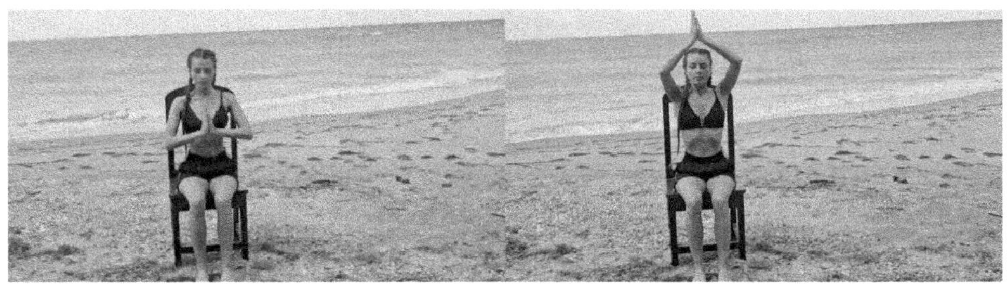

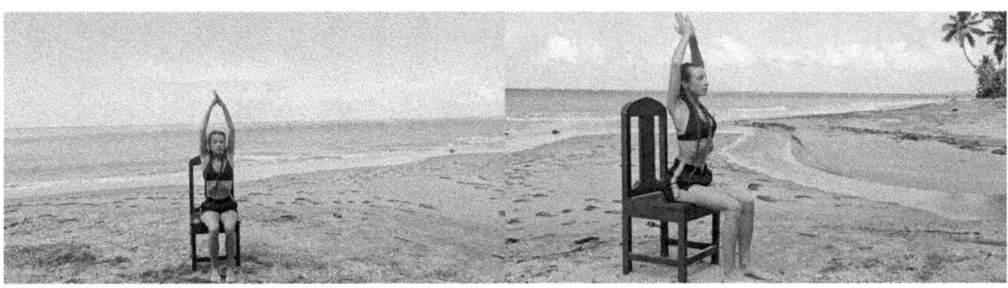

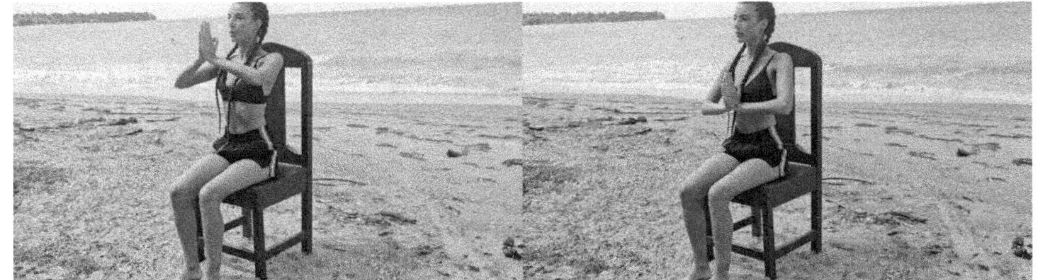

https://youtu.be/SK_Q5VLupV0

- Sit comfortably, hands at heart center.
- Inhale, raise the arms overhead.

- Exhale, lower the arms, bringing hands back to the heart center.
- Repeat for 5-10 cycles, syncing breath with movement.

Tip: Energize your body with each repetition, connecting breath and motion.

14. Seated Warrior II Pose

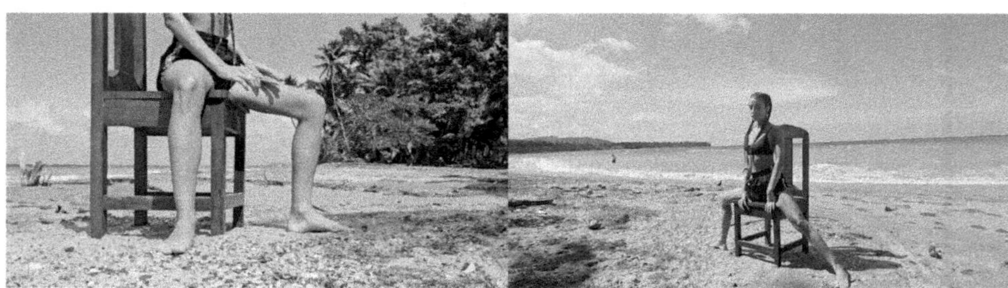

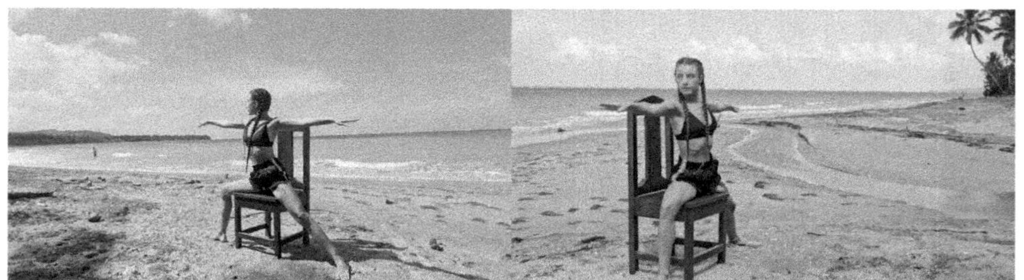

https://youtu.be/CYJClKDlYGU

- Sit on the chair with feet hip-width apart.
- Extend the right leg to the side, keeping the knee bent, toes pointing forward.
- Extend the left leg to the other side, keeping it straight, toes turned to point in front (same direction as the chair)

• Inhale, extend the arms to the side and parallel to the floor, palms facing down.

• Turn the head to gaze over the right fingertips.

• Hold for 20-30 seconds, feeling the stretch in the inner thigh.

• Return to the starting position and switch sides.

Tip: Engage the core, keep the spine straight, and maintain steady breath.

15. Chair Bridge Pose

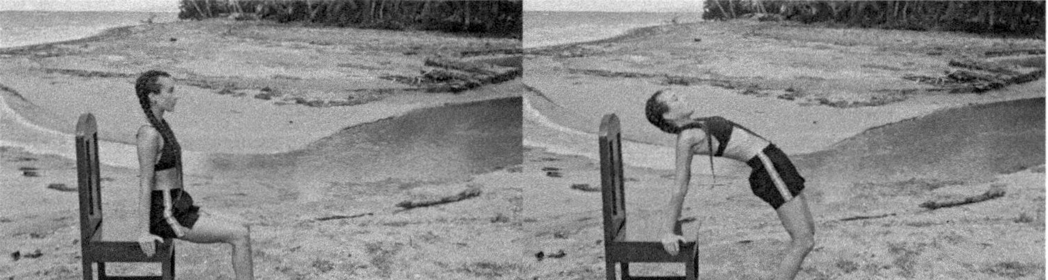

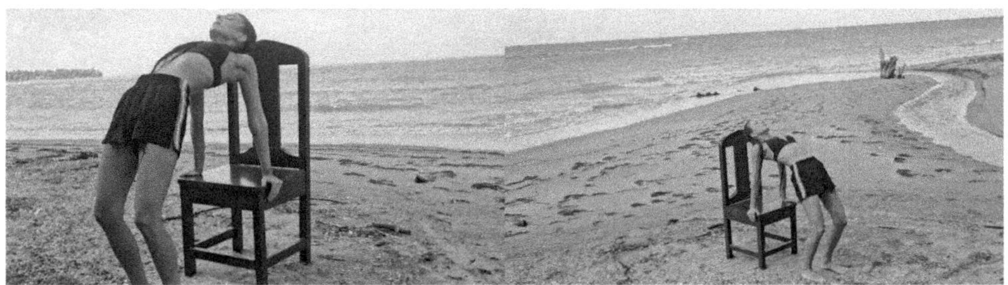

https://youtu.be/ghSeMpUrLoo

• Sit on the edge of the chair with feet flat, hip-width apart.

• Place your hands on the sides of the chair.

• Inhale, press through the hands, and lift the hips towards the ceiling (or sky).

• Hold for 15-20 seconds, engaging the glutes and core.

• Exhale and lower the hips back to the chair.

Tip: Keep the shoulders relaxed and focus on lifting through the hips.

16. Seated Revolved Triangle

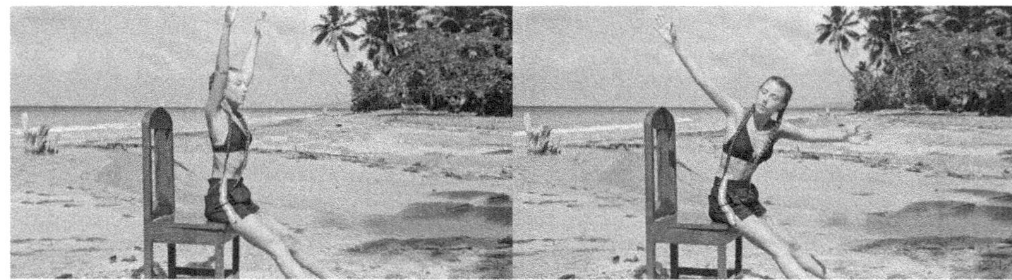

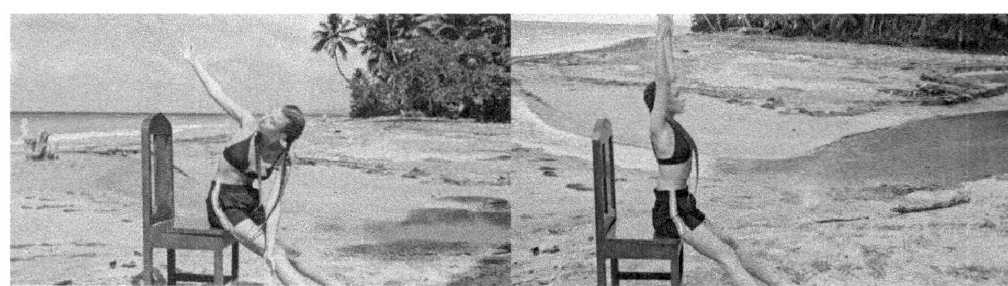

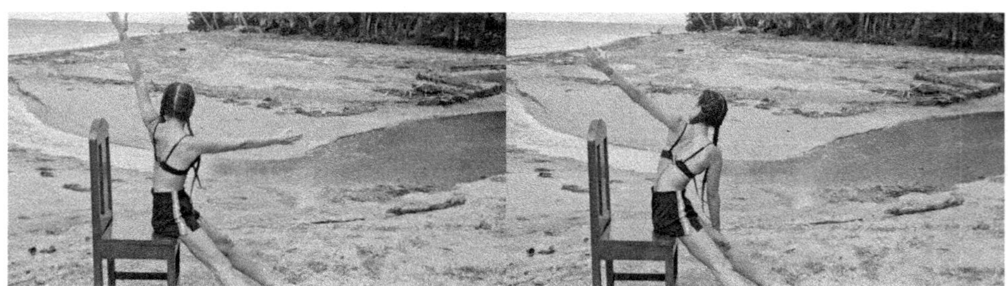

https://youtu.be/1-Ge5iNFCy0

- Sit tall with your legs extended.
- Inhale, lift the arms overhead.
- Exhale, twist to the right, bringing the left hand to the outside of the right leg.
- Reach the right arm behind, feeling a twist in the spine.
- Hold for 20-30 seconds, then switch sides.

Tip: Lengthen the spine with each inhale and deepen the twist with each exhale.

17. Inner Thigh Stretch

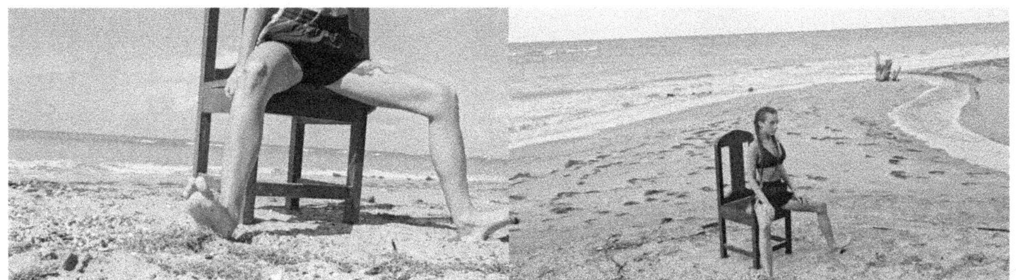

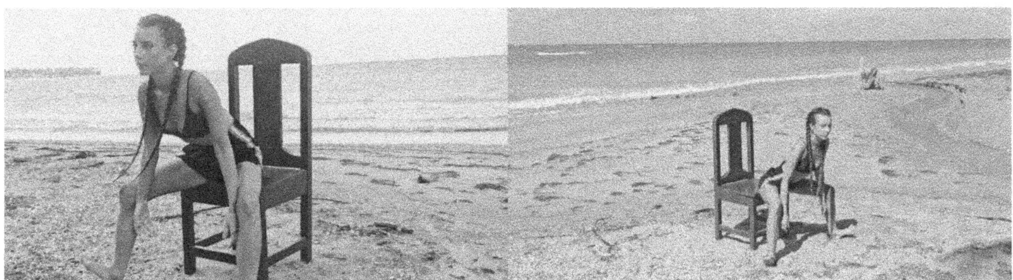

https://youtu.be/j5ONTVCTqUc

- Sit comfortably on the chair.
- Open the legs to the sides, toes pointing up.
- Inhale, lengthen the spine, and exhale, and hinge at the hips.
- Hold for 20-30 seconds, feeling the stretch in the inner thighs.

Tip: Keep the back straight and hinge from the hips for an effective stretch.

18. Seated Boat Pose

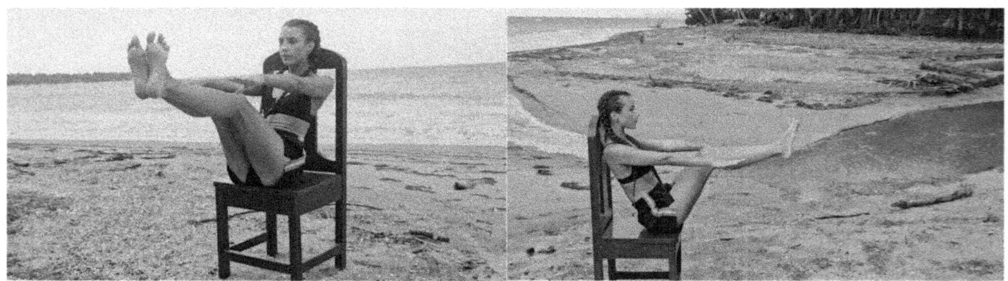

https://youtu.be/Mn1eYLNbcAY

- Sit at the edge of the chair with knees bent and feet flat.
- Inhale, lean back, lifting the feet off the floor.

- Extend the arms parallel to the floor.
- Hold for 15-20 seconds, engaging the core.
- Exhale and lower the feet back to the floor.

Tip: Keep the spine straight, chest lifted, and core engaged.

19. Seated Side Leg Lifts

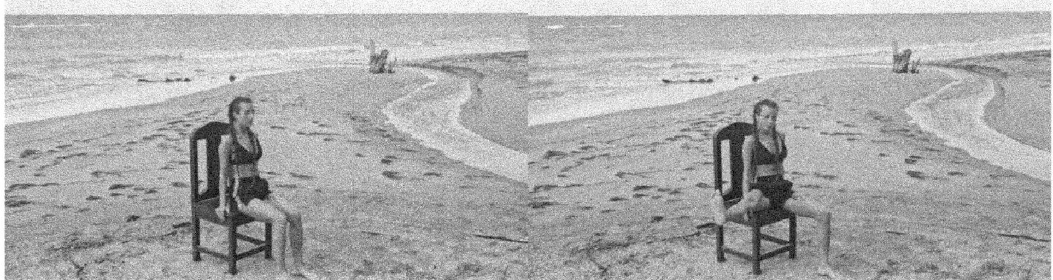

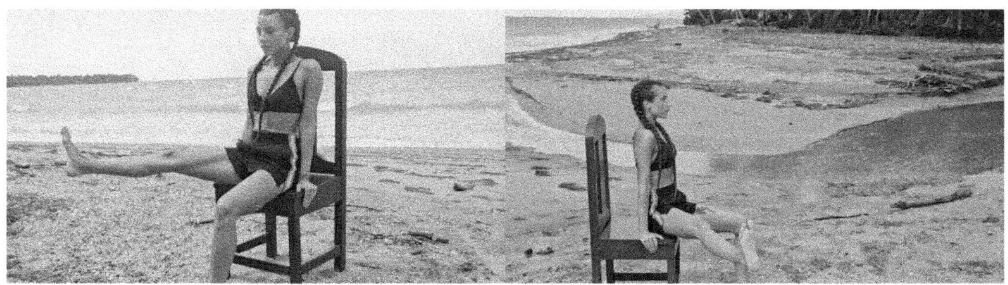

https://youtu.be/r2JoYRw603E

- Sit on the edge of the chair with hands gripping the sides.
- Lift the right leg to the side, keeping it straight.
- Hold for 10-15 seconds, feeling the engagement in the outer hip.
- Lower the leg and repeat on the other side.

Tip: Maintain a tall spine and engage the core for stability.

20. Chair Warrior III Pose

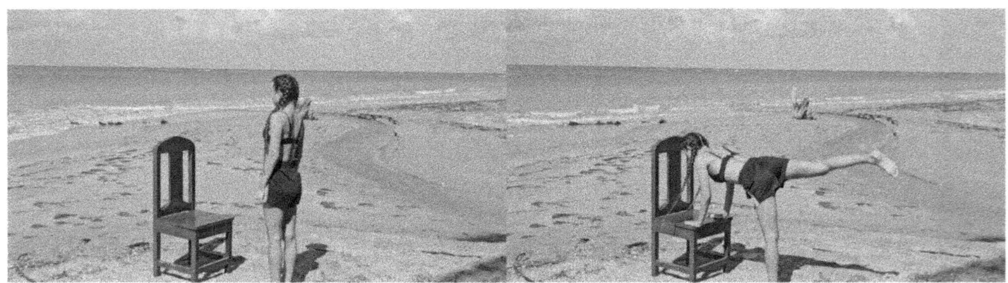

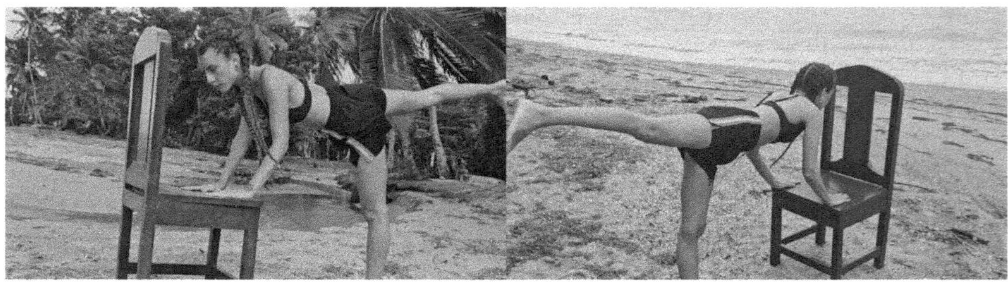

https://youtu.be/e5I3ZvTsvi8

- Stand facing the chair with feet flat on the floor/ground.
- Inhale, lift the right leg, extending it straight behind you.
- Simultaneously, lean the upper body forward, forming a straight line, and rest your hands on the chair, to support your balance.
- Hold for 15-20 seconds, engaging the core and extending through the lifted leg.
- Return to the starting position and switch sides.

Tip: Focus on balance, keeping the spine and lifted leg in alignment.

21. Quad Stretch

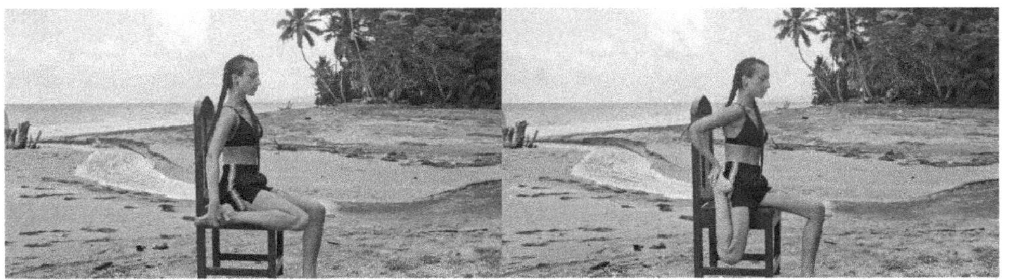

https://youtu.be/LYTbk82Pw-4

- Sit on the right side of the chair with feet hip-width apart.
- Bend the right knee, bringing the heel towards the right glute.
- Hold the right ankle with the right hand, feeling a stretch in the quad.
- Hold for 20-30 seconds, then switch sides.

Tip: Keep the knees close together and maintain an upright posture.

22. Chair Half-Moon Pose

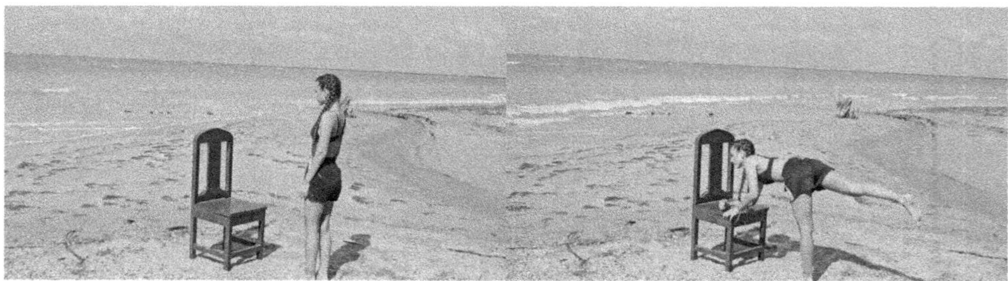

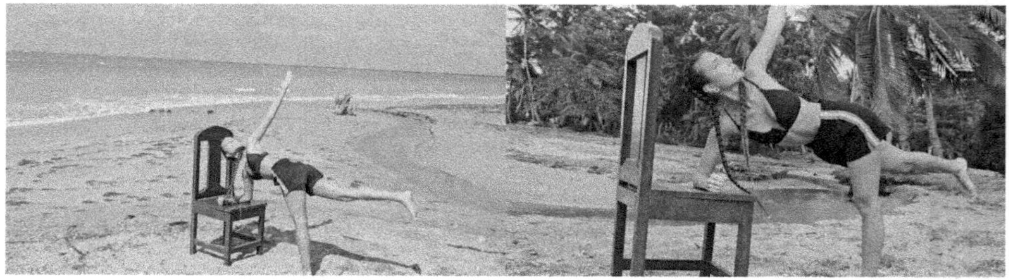

https://youtu.be/CFiz6TPdQFg

- Stand facing the chair with feet flat on the floor.
- Inhale, lean forward, placing your right elbow on the chair and simultaneously lift the right leg, extending it straight behind you.
- Lift the left hand towards the ceiling, twisting your torso.
- Hold for 15-20 seconds, engaging the core and extending through the lifted leg.
- Return to the starting position and switch sides.

23. Standing Figure 4 Stretch

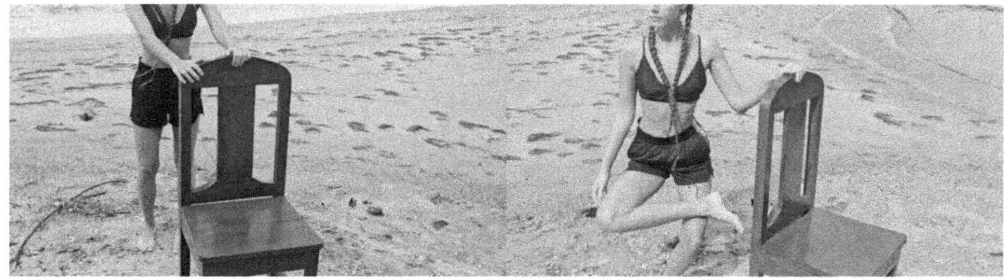

https://youtu.be/uk4T5jzLCBs

- Stand one step behind the chair, feet hip-width apart.
- Hold your hands on the backrest of the chair for support.
- Lift the right foot and cross it over the left thigh.
- Bend the left knee, sitting back into a "figure 4" position.
- Hold for 20-30 seconds, feeling the stretch in the outer hip.
- Switch sides and repeat.

Tip: Maintain balance by engaging the core and keeping the chest lifted.

24. Chair Frontal Plank

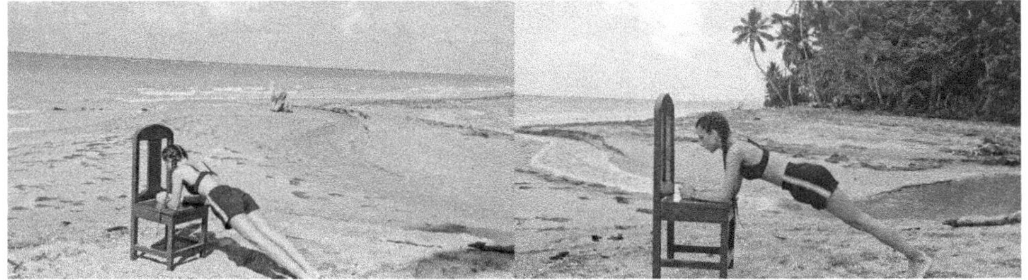

https://youtu.be/6MAyNHi8Q9Q

- Get into a plank position, with your elbows on the chair and your toes on the floor.
- Lift the hips, engaging your core, creating a straight line with your body.
- Hold for 15-20 seconds, engaging the abdominal muscles, the glutes and the thighs.

25. Seated Camel Pose

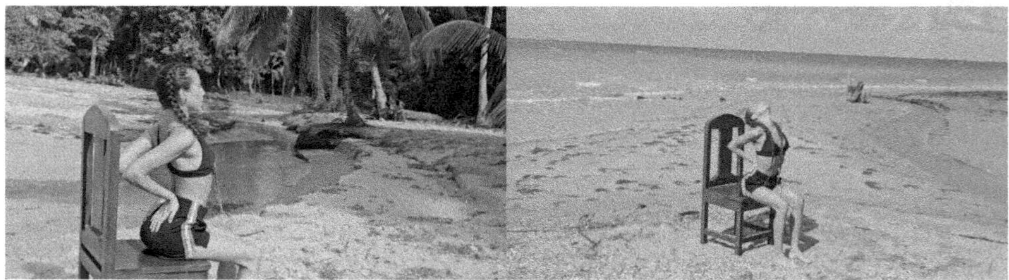

https://youtu.be/3hnPz8_zWSY

- Sit on the chair with knees bent and feet flat.
- Place hands on the lower back, fingers pointing down.

- Inhale, lift the chest, and arch the back.
- Hold for 15-20 seconds, feeling a stretch in the front of the body.

Tip: Keep the neck in a neutral position and focus on the opening of the chest.

Building Strength and Flexibility in Chair Yoga

Strength and flexibility in chair yoga is a dynamic process that transforms the body and mind. Let's explore the specific poses and strategies that will empower you to elevate your practice by focusing on building both strength and flexibility.

Strengthening with Seated Warrior III Pose:

Pose Modification: Begin with the Seated Warrior III Pose introduced earlier.

Advanced Variation: Gradually extend the arms forward while maintaining a straight back, intensifying the engagement of the core and lower back muscles.

Enhancing Flexibility with Quad Stretch:

Pose Modification: Start with the basic Quad Stretch described earlier.

Advanced Variation: While in the stretch, gently press the foot into the hand, increasing the depth of the stretch and promoting greater flexibility in the quadriceps.

Progressive Strength in Plank Positions:

Pose Modification: Begin with a Chair Plank for foundational strength.

Advanced Variation: Lift one leg off the ground while in the plank position, challenging your core stability and enhancing overall strength.

Deepening Flexibility in Seated Camel Pose:

Pose Modification: Practice the Seated Camel Pose as outlined.

Advanced Variation: While in the pose, extend one arm overhead and reach towards the opposite side, deepening the stretch along the front of the body.

Incorporate these modifications and variations into your chair yoga routine, gradually increasing the difficulty level. Remember, the key lies in consistent practice and listening to your body. As you progressively challenge yourself, you'll find the perfect balance between building strength and enhancing flexibility, creating a harmonious and transformative chair yoga practice.

Addressing Common Challenges at Intermediate Level

Yoga Plateaus: Breaking Through Stagnation

At the intermediate level, it's not uncommon to encounter plateaus where progress may seem stalled. Recognizing these plateaus is the first step to overcoming them.

Strategies to Break Through

Diversify Your Routine: Introduce new poses or variations to keep your practice fresh and challenging.

Set Micro-Goals: Break down larger goals into smaller, achievable milestones to reignite a sense of accomplishment.

Explore New Styles: Consider exploring different styles of yoga to provide a well-rounded challenge to your body and mind.

Poses Feel Too Challenging: Navigating Discomfort

As you advance, some poses may feel significantly more challenging. This discomfort is a natural part of growth but requires a thoughtful approach.

Strategies to Overcome

Modify Poses: Explore variations or use props to make challenging poses more accessible.

Consistent Practice: Regular, intentional practice gradually increases strength and flexibility, making challenging poses more attainable.

Mindful Breathing: Focus on steady breathing to calm the mind and release tension, allowing you to approach challenging poses with a centered mindset.

Poses Feel Too Simple: Finding Depth in Simplicity

Feeling that poses are too simple might arise as your body adapts to familiar movements. However, simplicity provides an opportunity for refinement.

Strategies to Deepen Your Practice

Mindful Alignment: Pay attention to the details of each pose, ensuring proper alignment and engagement.

Slow, Controlled Movements: Embrace slower transitions, allowing you to concentrate on the quality of each movement.

Mind-Body Connection: Build a connection between your breath and movements, bringing a meditative aspect to seemingly simple poses.

Struggling with Consistency

Maintaining a consistent practice can be challenging due to busy schedules, fatigue, or other life demands.

Strategies to Establish Consistency

Set Realistic Goals: Establish achievable, bite-sized goals to avoid feeling overwhelmed.

Create a Schedule: Dedicate specific time slots for your practice, making it a non-negotiable part of your routine.

Find Accountability: Share your progress in chair yoga with a friend or join a community to stay motivated and accountable.

Balancing Intensity

Finding the right balance between pushing your limits and avoiding overexertion is necessary for a sustainable practice.

Strategies to Maintain Balance

Listen to Your Body: Pay attention to signals of fatigue or discomfort and adjust your intensity accordingly.

Periodization: Incorporate higher and lower intensity periods to allow for recovery and prevent burnout.

Consult a Professional: If needed, seek guidance from a yoga instructor or healthcare professional to tailor your practice to your needs. Otherwise, this book is all you need.

These challenges are not roadblocks but stepping stones towards growth while being consistent with chair yoga. Embrace the ebb and flow of your practice, applying these strategies to face challenges, break plateaus, and find fulfillment both in the simplicity and complexity of chair yoga poses.

Weekly Planner for Continued Progress

Monday: Embracing the Foundation with Beginner Poses	Kickstart your week with a focus on foundational poses. These beginner poses provide a solid base for your practice, allowing you to concentrate on proper alignment and mindful breathing. Consider incorporating poses such as Seated Mountain Pose, Gentle Chair Twist, and Seated Cat-Cow. As you revisit these fundamental movements, pay attention to the subtleties, ensuring a strong connection between your breath and each pose.
Tuesday: Transitioning with Beginner-Intermediate Poses	As the week progresses, introduce a blend of beginner and intermediate poses to facilitate a smooth transition. Engage in poses like Seated Warrior I, Chair Pigeon Pose, and Seated Forward Bend with a slightly deeper exploration. This combination allows you to gradually challenge your body and build on the foundations laid on Monday. Focus on the fluidity of movements and the development of both strength and flexibility.
Wednesday: Elevating Your Practice with Intermediate Poses	Midweek is an excellent time to delve into more advanced variations of intermediate poses. Experiment with Seated Extended Triangle Pose, Chair High Lunge, and Seated Warrior III. These poses introduce heightened challenges to your stability and flexibility. Concentrate on maintaining a steady breath and refining your alignment. This day is an important point for growth as you make progress.
Thursday: Active Recovery and Mindful Reflection	Give your body a chance to recover with a day dedicated to active recovery. Engage in gentle movements like seated forward folds and neck stretches. This day also serves as an opportunity for mindful reflection. Revisit your goals, assess your progress, and celebrate the achievements, no matter how small. Acknowledge any challenges encountered during the week and plan adjustments for continued improvement.
Friday: Pushing Limits with Advanced Poses	As the weekend approaches, challenge yourself with a mix of advanced poses. Explore Upper Back Stretch, Seated Side Angle Pose and Compass Pose. This combination aims to push your limits, fostering increased strength and flexibility. Pay attention to the subtleties of each pose, ensuring a balanced and controlled execution.

Encouragement to Revisit Goals

Throughout the week, consistently revisit your goals. Reflect on the progress made, areas that need attention, and how your body responds to the challenges. Adjust your weekly planner accordingly, tailoring it to your needs and aspirations. Maintaining this routine empowers a sense of discipline and creates a path for continual progress while performing chair yoga.

Practical Knowledge: Remember to listen to your body and modify poses as needed. Consult a healthcare professional or yoga instructor if you encounter discomfort beyond the normal stretch. Incorporate warm-up and cool-down sessions to prepare your body and aid recovery. Consistency and patience are key to sustained progress.

Final Words

As we conclude our exploration of intermediate chair yoga poses, we must reflect on how far we have come in our chair yoga journey. Lee Haney's words, "Exercise to stimulate, not to annihilate," reverberate throughout this chapter, reminding us that progress is a gradual process, one pose at a time.

In exploring Seated Warrior III, Quad Stretches, and various other intermediate poses, we've aimed to provide you with the tools to stimulate growth in both strength and flexibility. The weekly planner is a practical guide to advance through poses systematically, ensuring a balanced and progressive practice.

Key Takeaways

Balancing Act: Intermediate chair yoga is a delicate balance between refining simplicity and facing the challenges of complexity. Each pose positively affects your progress, bringing a harmonious blend of strength and flexibility.

Consistency is Key: The weekly planner emphasizes the importance of consistent practice. Regular engagement with poses and mindful reflection pave the way for continuous improvement.

The next chapter **Step #6** awaits with a new set of challenges and triumphs. "Mastering Advanced Poses" will highlight the pinnacle of chair yoga practice. Uncover the secrets of poses that push the boundaries, testing your limits and unlocking new dimensions in your journey towards mastery. Embrace the challenge, stay committed, and let's elevate your chair yoga practice to new heights together.

Step #6: Mastering Advanced Poses

"Physical fitness is not only one of the most important keys to a healthy body, it is the basis of dynamic and creative intellectual activity." —John F. Kennedy.

Chair yoga offers a unique avenue for seniors to enhance physical fitness and promote overall health. We now focus on Chapter 6 to explore advanced poses. These poses are a bit challenging but provide an opportunity for further strengthening, flexibility, and balance. Remember, the essence lies in regularly performing and gradually mastering these poses. So, let's start with a commitment to improved wellness and vitality.

Unlocking Mastery: 18 Advanced Chair Yoga Poses for Senior Vitality

This section will discuss advanced chair yoga poses designed to improve your practice and promote vitality in your golden years. These poses are carefully selected to challenge and enhance your strength, flexibility, and balance, all while maintaining the accessibility and safety of chair yoga. Now, let's explore the first advanced pose.

1. *Chair pose (Utkatasana)*

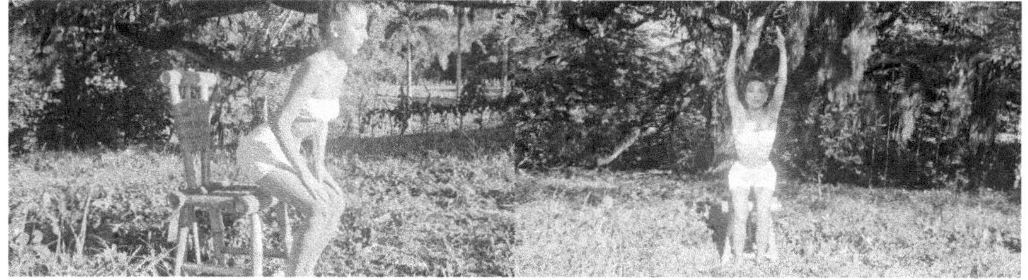

https://youtu.be/6H976UK5q1E

• Sit on the chair with your legs hip-width apart, and feet planted on the ground.

• Inhale as you lengthen your spine and gently lean forward.

• Exhale, as you bring your weight onto your feet, and slightly lift your hips off the chair, keeping your knees bent.

• Inhale as you lift your arms towards the sky.

• Maintain the posture for 20-30 seconds, then slowly return to a seated position.

Tip: Maintain a tall spine, and keep your knees behind the line of the toes.

2. Chair Cow Face Pose

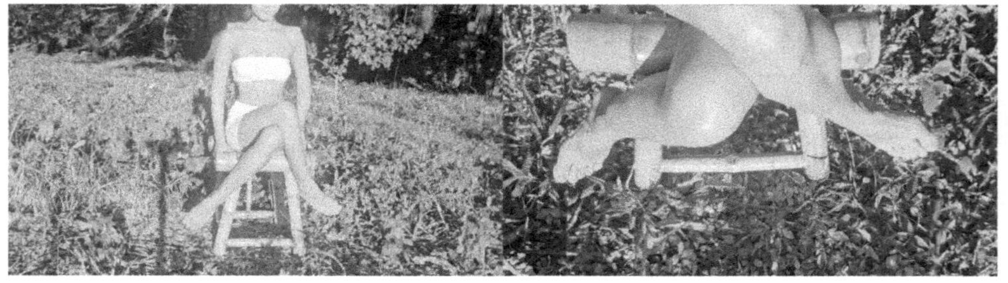

https://youtu.be/YsVgbqpeeD8

• Sit on the chair with your feet close together.

• Cross your right leg over your left leg, reaching the heel over the left chair leg.

• Stretch your left leg towards the right, reaching the right chair leg with your heel. You can use your hand to position it.

• Lengthen your back, and hold for 20-30 seconds.

• Return to the starting position and switch sides.

Tip: Reach the chair legs with your foot if your heel is too far. Bring your feet up on the chair for a deeper stretch.

3. Chair Wide-Legged Forward Bend

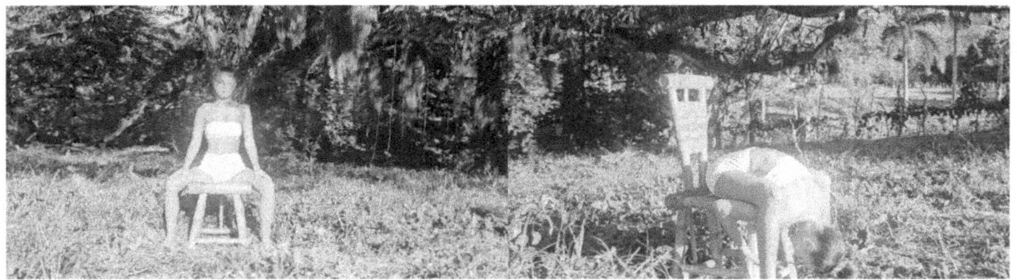

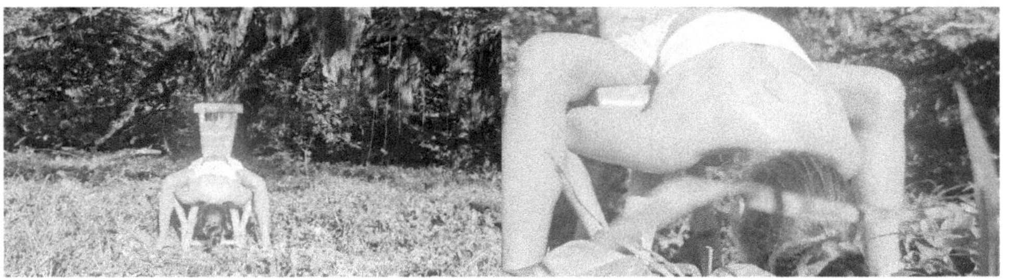

https://youtu.be/REBEYRXmkFQ

- Sit comfortably on the chair with your legs wide apart.
- Inhale, lengthen your spine, and as you exhale, hinge at your hips, reaching your hands towards the floor.
- Hold onto the chair legs, allowing your chest to come closer to your thighs.
- Feel a gentle stretch in your hamstrings and lower back.
- Hold for 20-30 seconds, and slowly return to an upright position.

Tip: Keep your back straight and focus on the sensation of lengthening through your spine.

4. *Advanced Eagle pose*

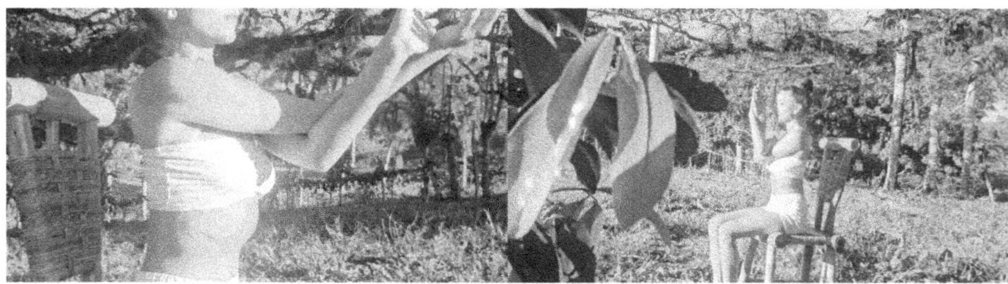

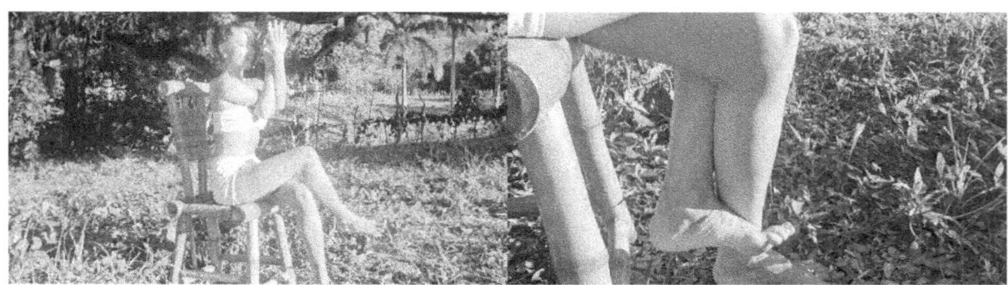

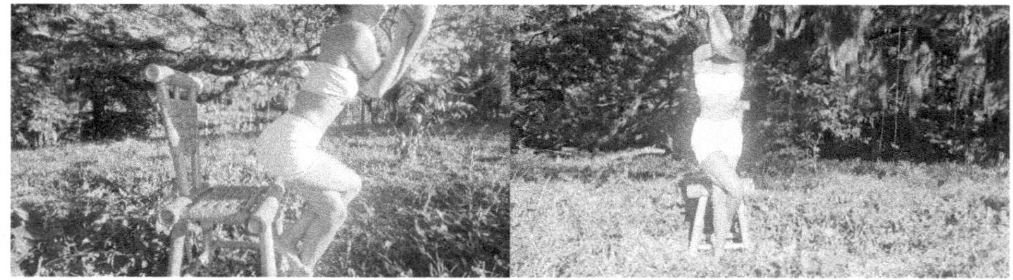

https://youtu.be/7ChQkxg7eCE

- Sit on the edge of the chair with feet flat on the ground.
- Inhale, extend arms to the sides.

• Exhale, cross the right arm over the left arm and lift the elbows while bringing the palms together.

• Inhale, lift your right leg, exhale, and cross it over the left leg, bringing the foot at the inner part of your left ankle.

• Lean forward, bringing your weight into your leg as inhaling, and lift your hips off your chair as exhaling.

• Hold for several breaths, then reverse all steps and repeat to the other side.

Tip: Keep your hips on the chair if standing up is challenging, and try to lift and sit back down several times to progress. To stretch more, stand up, straighten your legs, and lift the arms, while maintaining the pose.

5. Lotus Pose

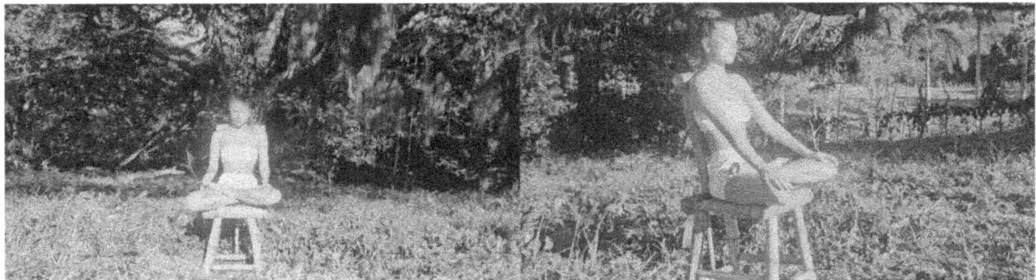

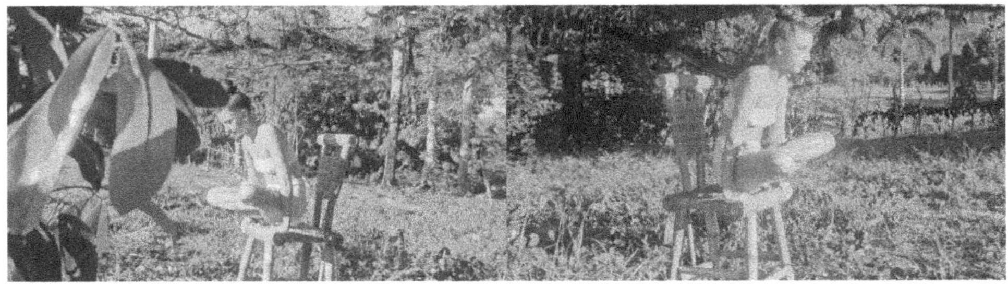

https://youtu.be/PxrjNG-7Yp8

• Start in a comfortable seated position on the chair.

• Cross your right ankle over your left thigh and bring your left ankle over your right thigh.

• Allow your knees to drop towards the floor gently.

• Find a comfortable position for your hands, either on your knees or in a mudra.

• Hold for a few breaths, feeling a stretch in your hips.

Tip: If Lotus Pose is too challenging, opt for Half Lotus or simply cross your legs comfortably. If you want to challenge yourself more, try Floating Lotus by holding the sides of the chair with your hands and lifting the hips holding your weight into your hands.

6. Chair Splits Prep

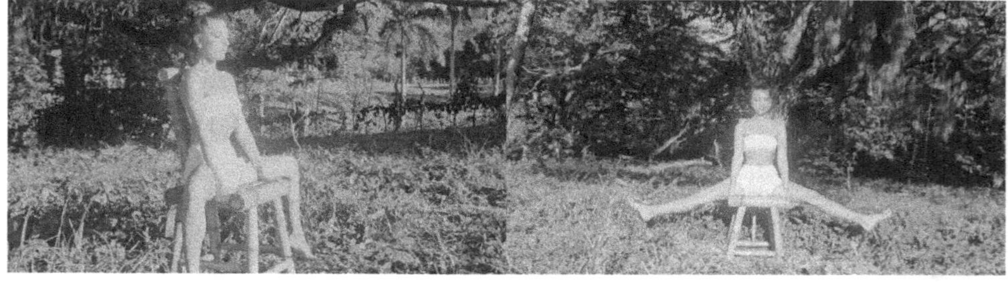

https://youtu.be/Xzff9DFausw

• Sit on the chair with your legs feet wide apart.

• Open your legs wide to the sides.

• Grab the sides of the chair with your hands between the inner parts of your thighs.

• Inhale, elongate your spine, and exhale as you strengthen your legs, lifting the feet off the ground.

• Hold the pose for a few breaths, feeling the stretch in your inner thighs.

• Slowly return to an upright position.

Tip: Help by pushing with your hands to open your legs to the sides farther, in order to progress.

7. Extended Hands-to-Big-Toe Pose

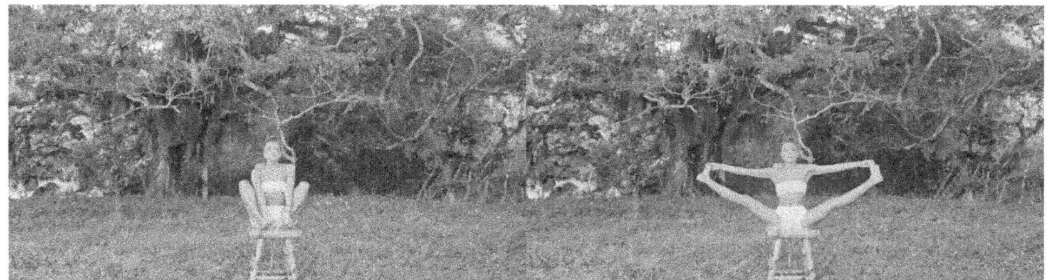

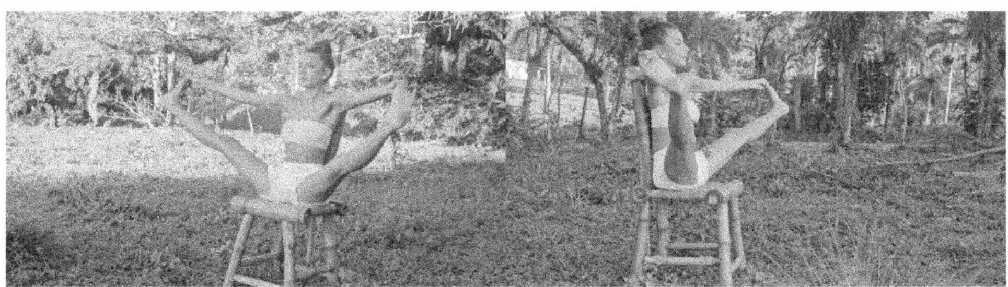

https://youtu.be/H_3onZmYCKw

- Sit at the edge of the chair with your feet hip wide apart.
- Lean back, lift both legs bringing the knees towards your chest, and hold the big toes with your hands.
- Straighten your legs to the sides, keeping your back straight.
- Hold for 15-20 seconds, then release.

Tip: If straightening the legs is too challenging, keep your knees bent and gradually progress into a more straightened position.

8. *Seated Side Angle Pose (Utthita Parsvakonasana)*

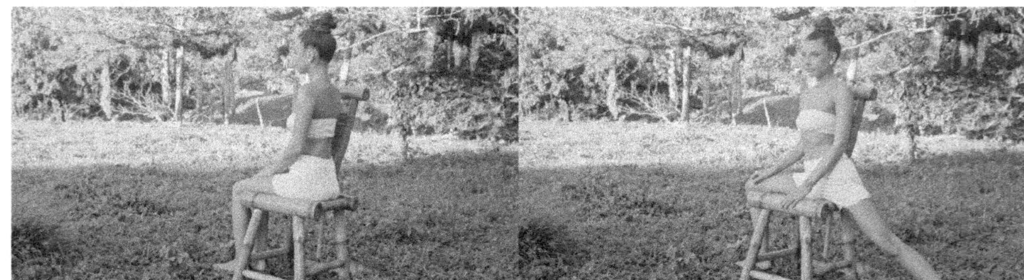

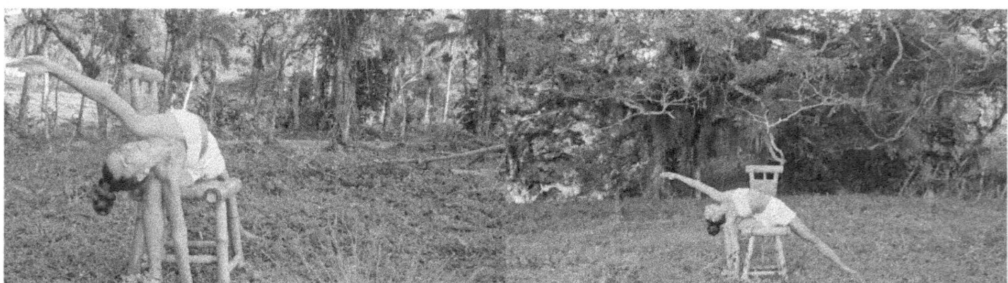

https://youtu.be/DbZ1denDVZY

- Sit with your right side close to the backrest of the chair with your feet flat on the ground.
- Extend your left leg straight back.
- Twist your torso to face front, and reach the ground with your right hand, bringing your right shoulder in front of your right knee.
- Turn your head to look towards the sky, and lift your left arm, forming a straight line with your left leg.
- Hold for 20-30 seconds, then return to the center and repeat on the other side.

Tip: Use the backrest of the chair to help get into the posture.

9. Chair Lord of the Fishes (Matsyndrasana)

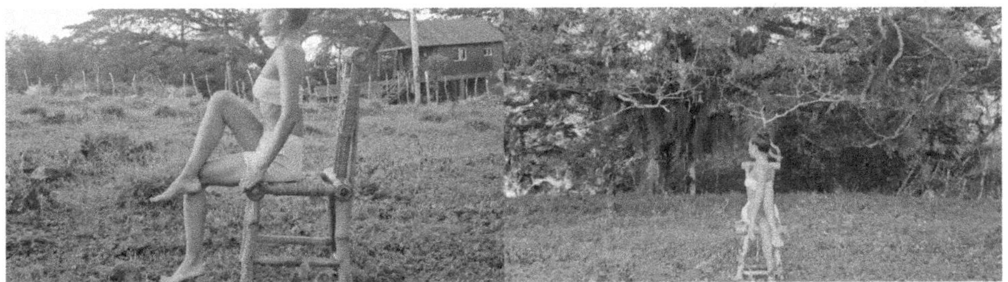

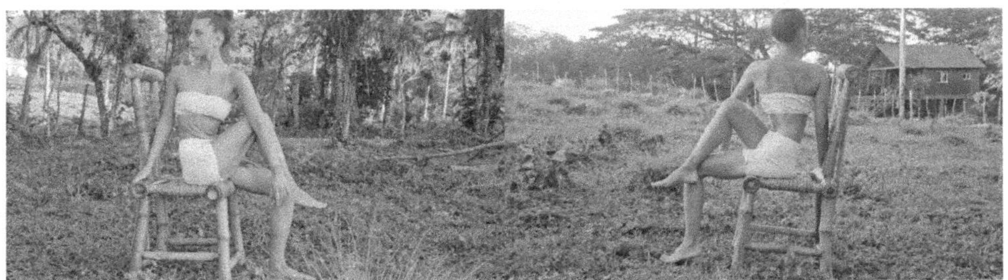

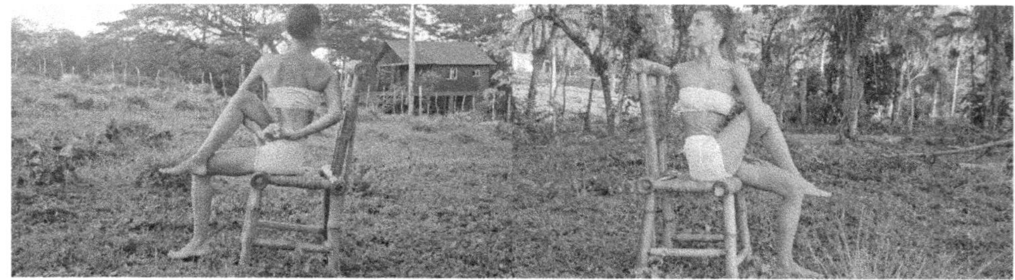

https://youtu.be/na-cSlvbns8

• Sit at the edge of the chair with your feet close together.

• Lift your right leg, bringing the ankle on the outside of your left knee.

• Inhale, lengthen your spine, and as you exhale, twist to the right bringing your left elbow to the outside of your right knee.

• You can stop here, at Half Lord of the Fishes, or continue by crossing your left hand under the right knee, and grabbing it with your right hand.

• Hold the pose for 20-30 seconds, then return to the starting position and repeat on the other side.

Tip: Focus on keeping a straight back. If you can't reach the elbow on the outside of your lifted knee, push your knee with your hand, and gradually progress into the pose.

10. Upper Back Stretch

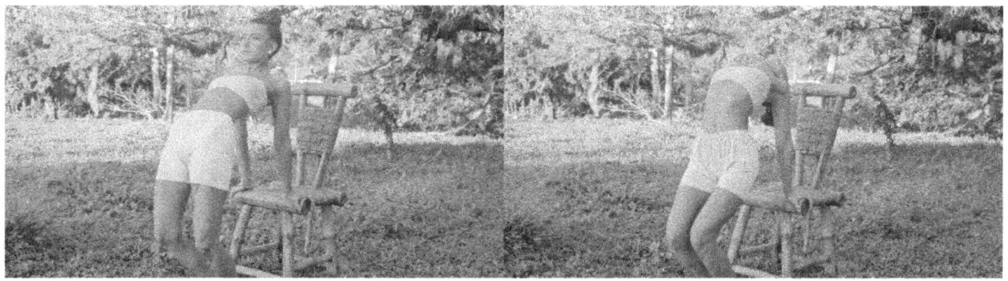

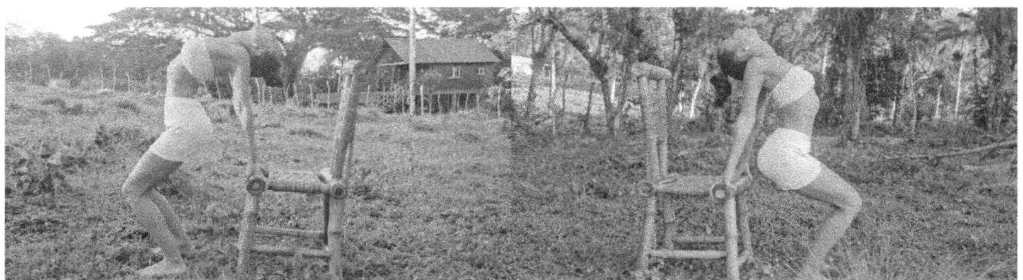

https://youtu.be/ZoeGr372GOk

- Stand in front of the chair, with your back to the chair.
- Lean backward to reach the seat of your chair with your hands.
- Inhale, lift your chest, arch your back, and let your neck fall behind.
- Exhale, push your hips down bending your knees while keeping your chest lifted and your arms straight.
- Hold for 20-30 seconds, then slowly return to an upright position.

Tip: Concentrate on lifting your chest as high as possible while simultaneously lowering your hips down.

11. Shoulders Stretch

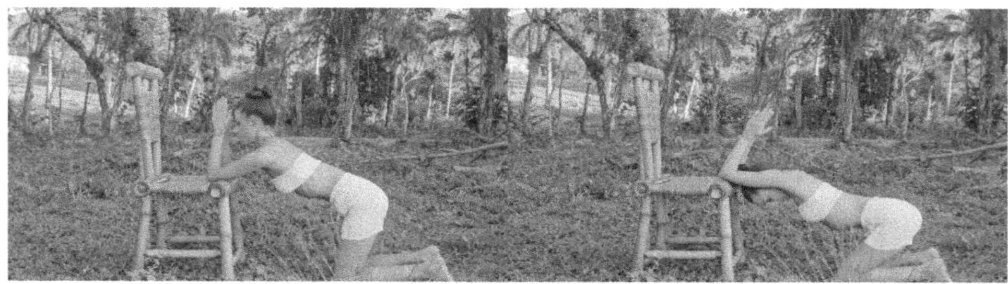

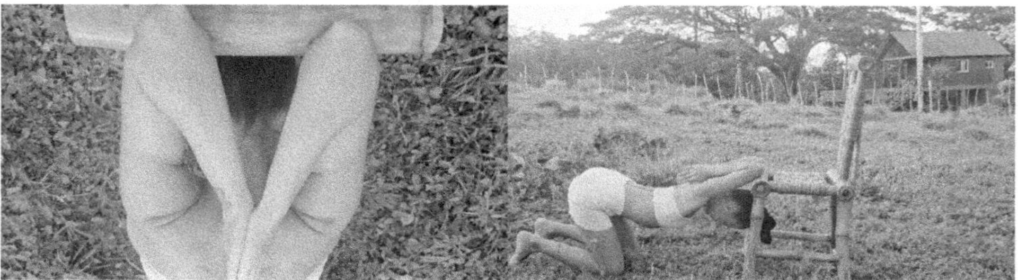

https://youtu.be/IqfNmMbPixk

• Start standing on your knees facing the chair, about one step behind.

• Lean forward, and reach the edge of your chair with your elbows.

• Bring your palms together, and bend your hips, lowering your head towards the ground, and bringing your hands close to your back.

• Hold for 20-30 seconds, feeling the stretch into your shoulders and upper arms.

Tip: Focus on maintaining a straight spine, and push into your elbows for extended stretch.

12. Chair Camel Pose (Ustrasana)

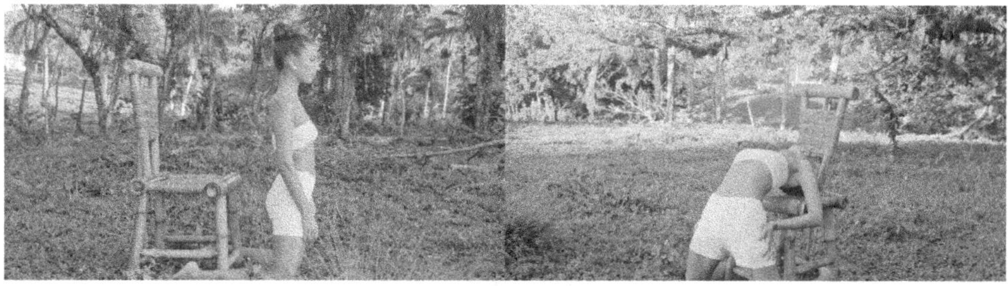

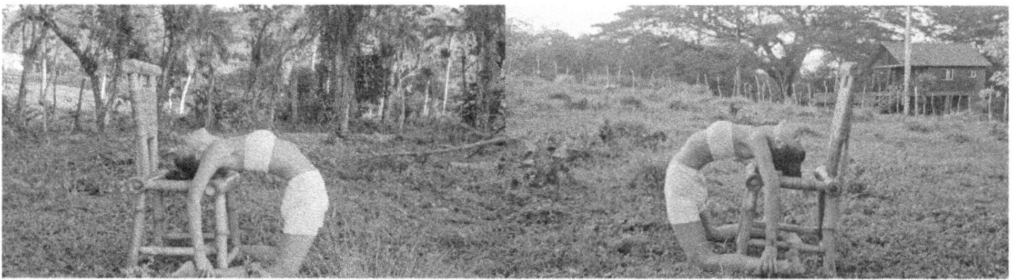

https://youtu.be/GbML920KVIg

- Start standing on your knees in front of your chair, with your feet close to the inner or outer sides of your chair, hip-width apart if possible.
- Inhale, lift your chest, and as you exhale, lean backward reaching your head on the chair.
- Push your hips forward, and grab your ankles with your hands.
- Hold the pose for a few breaths, then push into your ankles and raise your body up.

Tip: If you can't reach the chair with your head, reach it with your hands or elbows. Use a pillow under your knees if the floor is uncomfortable.

13. Chair Dancer Pose (Nataranjasana)

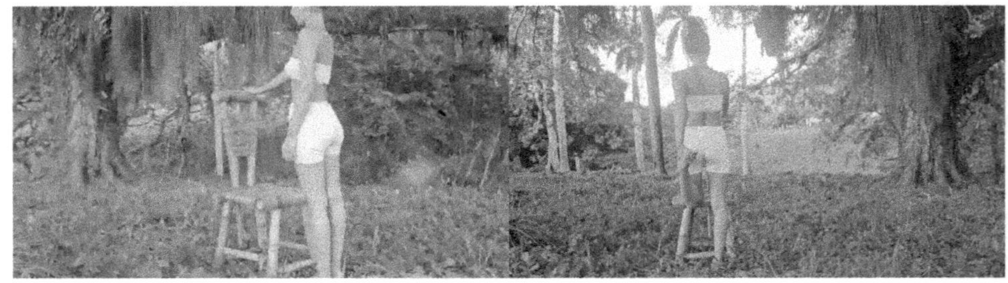

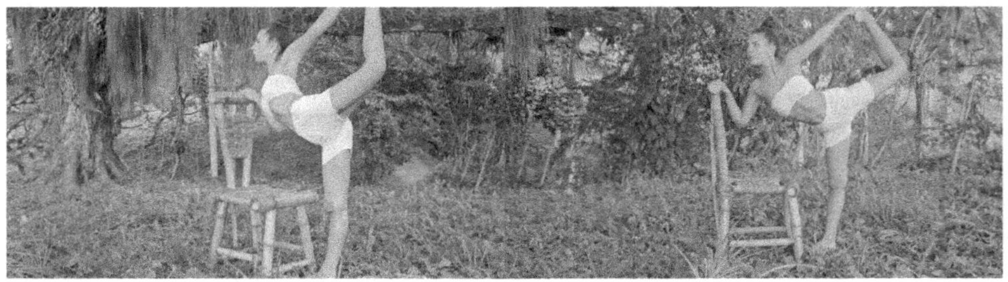

https://youtu.be/o_opkF_K4kM

• Stand facing the chair, with your right hand on the backrest of the chair.

• Lift your left foot towards your glutes, and hold it with your left hand.

• Inhale, lengthen your spine, and lift your chest.

• Exhale, lean forward and simultaneously lift your left leg together with your left hand towards the sky.

• Hold for 20-30 seconds, then return to the center and switch sides.

Tip: Engage your core and keep your gaze focused for better balance. If you can't reach your foot use a belt or a scarf. If you want to challenge yourself even more, try to lift the arm off the backrest of the chair.

14. Chair Lizard Pose

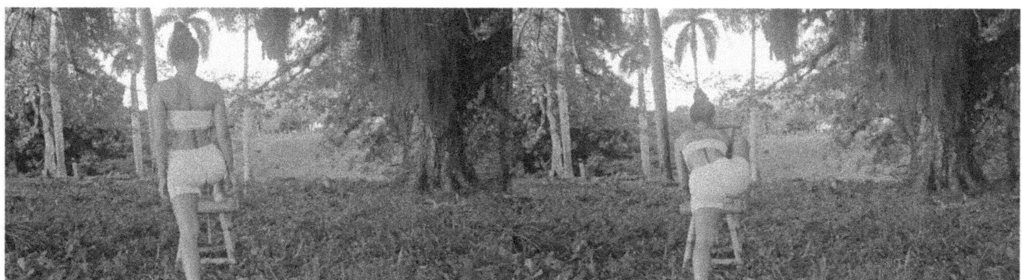

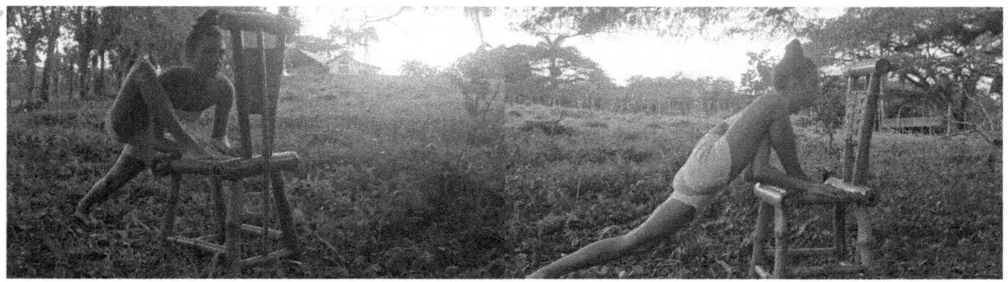

https://youtu.be/IWNMXDECBo8

• Stand facing the chair, about two steps away.

• Inhale, lift your right foot, and place it on the sit of the chair, making a big step.

• Exhale, lengthen your spine, and lean forward, placing your hands and your bent elbows on the chair.

• Your right shoulder must be either under or next to your right knee.

• Hold for 20-30 seconds feeling the deep stretch into your hips and thighs.

• Return to the center and repeat on the other side.

Tip: Focus on maintaining a straight back, and keep your neck aligned with your spine.

15. Seated Compass Pose

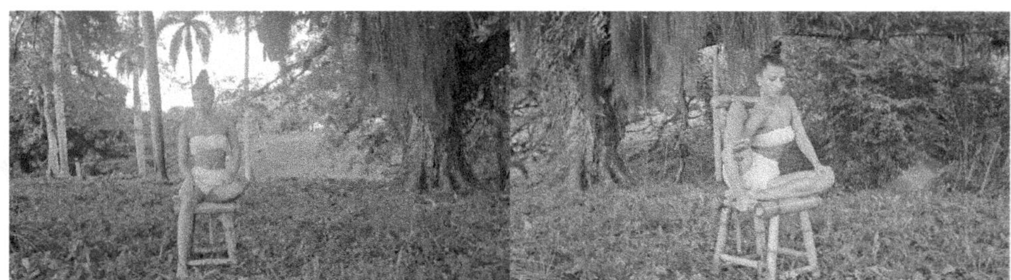

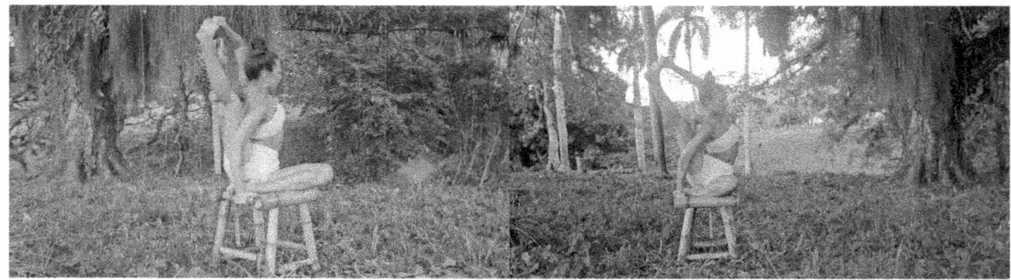

https://youtu.be/nXuqZHDOBok

• Seat on the chair with your left foot under your right hip.

• Bring your weight into your left hip.

• Lift your right leg, and reach the right side of the chair with your left hand, placing your upper arm under the right knee.

• Grab your right foot with your left arm, and lift your leg straight, switching your torso to the left.

• Position your head outside of your lifted hand.

• Hold for 20-30 seconds, feeling the stretch into your hamstrings, side body, and shoulders.

• Return to the center, and repeat on the other side.

Tip: Modify the stretch based on your flexibility, avoiding any discomfort. Use a scarf or a belt if necessary.

16. Seated Crow Pose (Kakasana prep.)

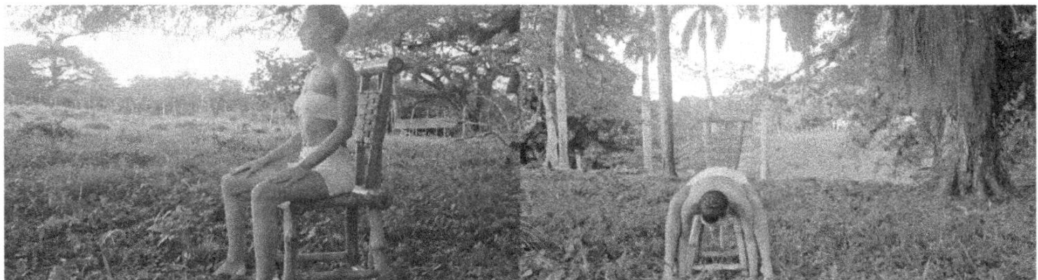

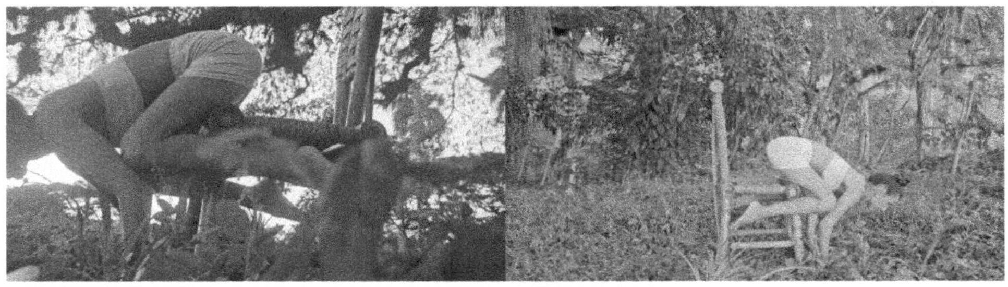

https://youtu.be/AbloeskMPKw

• Begin by sitting on the chair with your knees bent and legs opened to the sides, feet pointing front.

• Inhale, lengthen your spine, and as you exhale, lean forward, reaching your hands on the ground, next to your legs, fingers pointing forward.

• Bring your weight onto your hands, slightly lifting your hips, and position your knees on your upper arms lifting your feet off the ground.

• Hold for 20-30 seconds, and slowly return to an upright position.

Tip: Focus on holding your weight mostly onto your hands.

17. L-sit Prep (Brahmacharyasana)

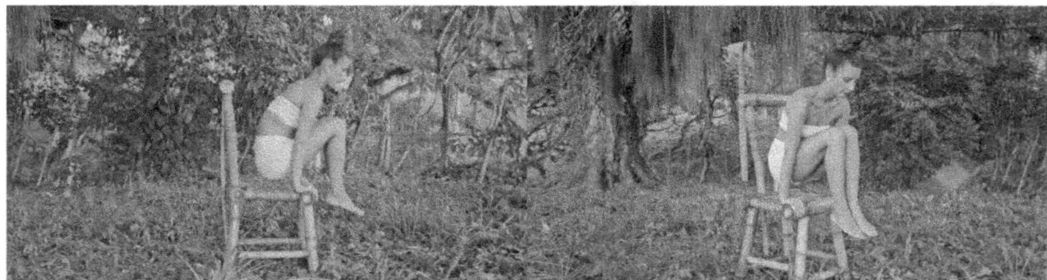

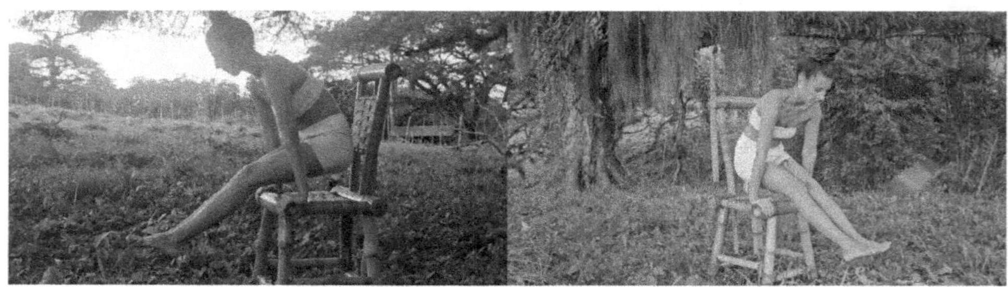

https://youtu.be/whqG8g6x9IA

• Begin seated, hands on the chair, fingers pointing forward.

• Lift your legs off the ground, bringing your knees towards your chest.

• Shift your weight onto your hands, finding balance on the chair.

• Engage your core and hold the position, gradually extending your legs if comfortable.

• To release, lower your feet back to the ground and sit back down.

Tip: Start with small lifts and gradually progress as your strength and confidence grow.

18. Butterfly Pose (Baddha Konasana)

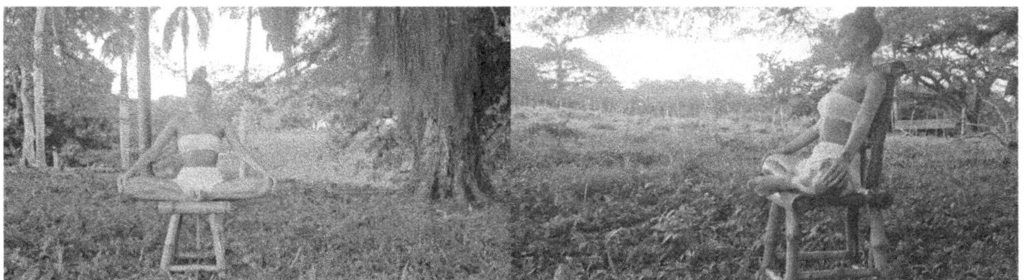

https://youtu.be/1tGTMxae6jk

• Sit tall on the chair, with feet flat on the ground.

• Bring your knees towards your chest, placing your feet on the chair.

• Join your soles together and position them close to your pelvis.

• Inhale, lengthen your spine, and as you exhale, press your knees down with your hands, feeling a stretch in your inner thighs.

• Hold the pose for 20-30 seconds, then release.

Tip: Focus on keeping your spine straight, use a pillow under your hips for better comfort.

Incorporating Flow and Fluidity in Movements

Embracing the fluidity of movements in your chair yoga routine can be a game-changer, offering physical benefits and a sense of satisfaction in your practice. Achieving a seamless flow might seem challenging for beginners, but with dedication and these practical tips, you'll elevate your chair yoga experience to new heights. (Life, n.d.)

Tips for Adding Flow and Fluidity

Mindful Transitions: Focus on the transitions between poses. Move deliberately, paying attention to the sensations in your body. Connect each movement with your breath, allowing the inhales and exhales to guide your flow.

Create Sequences: Design simple sequences that naturally flow from one pose to the next. For example, moving from a seated twist to a gentle forward bend creates a harmonious sequence.

Smooth Breath Integration: Coordinate your breath with movements. Inhale during expansive poses and exhale during compressive ones. Smooth, controlled breathing fosters a sense of calm and helps to synchronize your movements.

Explore Circularity: Introduce circular motions into your routine. For instance, circle your wrists and shoulders or gently rotate your spine. Circular movements enhance flexibility and promote a sense of fluidity.

Embrace Modifications: Modify poses to create a continuous flow that suits your comfort and ability. Feel free to adapt movements, emphasizing the flow's essence rather than strictly adhering to traditional poses.

Play with Rhythm: Experiment with the pace of your movements. Flow doesn't have to be fast; a slow and deliberate rhythm can be equally beneficial. Adjust the tempo to match your energy level and mood for the day.

Smooth Transitions Between Sides: When working on asymmetrical poses, maintain a seamless transition from one side to the other. This helps maintain balance and ensures both sides of your body receive equal attention.

Listen to Your Body: Pay close attention to how your body responds to each movement. If a transition feels challenging, approach it patiently and modify it as needed.

By incorporating these tips into your chair yoga routine, you'll enhance the fluidity of your movements and experience the joy of a more seamless practice.

Advanced Meditation and Breathing Techniques

As you delve deeper into your chair yoga practice, advanced meditation and intricate breathing techniques can become powerful tools for reaching a heightened sense of mindfulness and inner balance. Here are some advanced practices to supplement chair yoga. (*4 Advanced Meditation Techniques and Tools to Deepen Your Practice*, 2019)

Advanced Meditation Tools

Body Scan Meditation: Shift your focus systematically through different parts of your body, bringing awareness to each area. This technique promotes relaxation, heightened body awareness, and a sense of unity between mind and body.

Loving-Kindness Meditation (Metta): Extend your meditation beyond personal fitness to develop love and compassion for yourself and others. Use phrases like "May I be happy, may I be healthy," fostering a sense of interconnectedness.

Mantra Meditation: Select a mantra that resonates with you and repeat it silently or aloud during meditation. Mantras can be words, sounds, or phrases as a focal point for meditation.

Visualization Meditation: Envision peaceful scenes or scenarios during meditation, engaging your senses. Visualization can enhance relaxation, creativity, and a deeper connection with your inner self.

Transcendental Meditation (TM): Learn a personalized mantra from a certified TM teacher and use it for 15-20 minutes twice a day. Transcendental Meditation (TM) is renowned for its simplicity and efficacy in inducing profound relaxation and heightened awareness.

Intricate Breathing Techniques

Nadi Shodhana (Alternate Nostril Breathing): Close one nostril and inhale deeply through the other, then close the inhaling nostril and exhale through the opposite side. This technique balances the energy flow in your body and enhances mental clarity.

Kapalabhati (Skull Shining Breath): Rapidly exhale short bursts of breath through your nose, followed by passive inhalations. Kapalabhati energizes the body, clears the mind, and improves lung capacity.

Bhramari (Bee Breath): Inhale deeply through your nose and exhale slowly while humming like a bee. Bhramari calms the mind, reduces stress, and promotes a sense of tranquility.

Ujjayi Breath (Victorious Breath): Inhale deeply through your nose, constricting the back of your throat, creating an oceanic sound. Ujjayi breathing enhances concentration, warms the body, and promotes a meditative state.

Sitali (Cooling Breath): Inhale through a rolled tongue or pursed lips, exhale through the nose. Sitali cools the body, reduces stress, and enhances a sense of calmness.

Gradually integrate these advanced meditation tools and breathing techniques into your chair yoga routine. Remember to maintain a gentle and mindful approach as you explore these practices.

Weekly Challenges: Igniting Progress in Chair Yoga

Consider incorporating the following weekly challenges to infuse excitement and challenge into your chair yoga routine. These challenges enhance strength, flexibility, and mindfulness, permitting steady progress.

Balance Booster Challenge:	Incorporate one new balance pose into your routine each day. This could include Seated Tree Pose, Seated Crow Pose, or any other balance-focused variation. Benefits: Enhances stability, concentration, and overall body awareness.
Extended Flow Challenge:	Design a chair yoga flow sequence comprising 10-15 poses. Practice the sequence thrice weekly, focusing on smooth transitions and steady breathing. Benefits: Improves movement fluidity, enhances cardiovascular health, and deepens your understanding of pose connections.
Mindful Meditation Challenge:	Dedicate 10 minutes daily to an advanced meditation technique such as Body Scan, Loving-Kindness, or Mantra Meditation. Benefits: Improves mindfulness, reduces stress, and promotes a deeper connection with your inner self.
Breath Mastery Challenge:	Explore a different intricate breathing technique daily, dedicating 5-10 minutes to practice. Rotate through Nadi Shodhana, Kapalabhati, Bhramari, Ujjayi Breath, and Sitali. Benefits: Enhances respiratory function, calms the nervous system, and improves breath control.
Progressive Stretch Challenge:	Select a specific muscle group (e.g., hips, shoulders, or spine) and focus on its flexibility throughout the week. Incorporate targeted stretches and observe your progress. Benefits: Increases flexibility, reduces muscle tension, and provides a tangible measure of improvement.

Remember to approach these challenges with a sense of curiosity and self-compassion. Progress in yoga is a personal venture, and these challenges are designed to add variety and stimulation to your practice.

Final Words

Quoting the wisdom of John F. Kennedy, "Physical fitness is not only one of the most important keys to a healthy body, it is the basis of dynamic and creative intellectual activity." As we bring this chapter to a close, let these words echo as a reminder of the profound link between physical well-being and intellectual vitality.

Throughout this chapter, we explored a repertoire of advanced chair yoga poses, unlocking the door to enhanced strength, flexibility, and balance. From the Seated Crow Pose, challenging our arm balance, to the Seated Lotus Pose, inviting us into a serene state, each pose has contributed to the richness of our chair yoga journey.

Key Takeaways

Progress is gradual: Mastering advanced poses is not about achieving perfection overnight. It's incremental progress where the onus is on the mindful exploration of each pose, appreciating the improvements along the way.

Challenge Enhances Growth: Embracing challenges, whether in balance, meditation, or breathing techniques, adds a layer of richness to your chair yoga practice. These challenges become stepping stones toward greater physical and mental resilience.

As we conclude this chapter, get ready for an exciting next step in your chair yoga adventure. Chapter 7 awaits with "The 28-Day Challenge," where we'll begin a transformative month-long practice, exploring the depth of chair yoga and embracing a holistic approach to better health. Get ready to set intentions, meet challenges head-on, and witness the evolution of your chair yoga practice.

Step #7: The 28-Day Challenge

"To enjoy the glow of good health, you must exercise." —Gene Tunney.

We often find ourselves standing at the crossroads of intention and action to achieve vibrant health. The timeless wisdom in Gene Tunney's words resonates profoundly, reminding us that the journey to wellness begins with a commitment to exercise. This chapter presents a transformative 28-Day Challenge, a roadmap that takes you from the starting point of chair yoga to a position of confidence and accomplishment. The exercises outlined in the following pages are designed to be your companions, guiding you through each step with clarity and simplicity. This challenge isn't just about moving; it's about progression, building confidence in your practice, and setting the stage for continued success. The next 28 days will be a dynamic exploration of your body's capabilities, laying the foundation for sustained fitness. So, without further ado, let's begin.

28 Days to Yoga Bliss:
« Your Chair Yoga Transformation »

Begin this transformative process as we guide you through 28 days of chair yoga, building a foundation of strength and flexibility. This unique guide ensures inclusivity, providing alternatives for all levels. We'll infuse zest into your practice by seamlessly blending familiar poses with new ones, keeping the routine dynamic and engaging. Each day's sequence takes just 10 minutes or less, making it accessible for even the busiest schedules. Let's dive into each week, discovering the benefits of every pose and unlocking the potential for a healthier, happier you.

Week 1: Foundations and Warm-Up

Day 1-2: Establishing the Basics

Gentle Neck and Shoulder Stretches:

- Begin by sitting comfortably in your chair.
- Inhale deeply, and as you exhale, gently tilt your head to one side, feeling a soothing stretch along your neck.
- Hold for a few breaths, then switch to the other side.
- Repeat this process for five breaths on each side.

These gentle neck and shoulder stretches alleviate tension, promoting flexibility and relieving discomfort. Please refer back to the video links we provided in the previous chapters for added clarity on the poses if you need a refresher.

Mindful Breathing Exercises:

Find a quiet moment to focus on your breath.

- Inhale deeply through your nose, counting to four, allowing your lungs to fill with air.
- Exhale slowly through your mouth, counting to six, releasing any tension.
- Repeat this process for ten breath cycles.

This mindful breathing exercise calms the mind, enhances concentration, and encourages a sense of inner peace.

Introduction to Foundational Poses:

Like in Step #2, explore foundational poses like the Seated Mountain Pose.

- Sit tall in your chair with your hands resting on your thighs.
- Inhale, lift your arms overhead, and bring them back down as you exhale.

This simple yet effective pose helps establish good posture, engages core muscles, and creates a sense of grounding and stability.

Day 3-5: Upper Body Warm-Up

Focus on Arms, Wrists, and Hands (Seated Arm Circles):

Activate your upper body with Seated Arm Circles.

• Extend your arms to the sides, palms facing down.

• Rotate your arms in small circles for 30 seconds, then reverse the direction.

This exercise improves circulation, warms up the shoulders, and reduces stiffness in the arms, wrists, and hands.

Slow Introduction to Seated Twists (Seated Twist):

Engage your core with Seated Twist.

• Sit straight, inhale, lengthen your spine, and exhale as you twist gently to one side.

• Hold the twist for 15 seconds, feeling the stretch.

• Repeat on the other side.

This exercise enhances spinal flexibility, massages internal organs, and makes your spine healthy.

Incorporating Fluid Movements (Seated Cat-Cow Stretch):

Combine breath with movement in a Seated Cat-Cow Stretch.

• Inhale, arching your back (Cow); exhale, rounding your spine (Cat).

• Repeat for 1 minute, allowing your breath to guide the fluidity of movement.

This exercise strengthens the core, promotes spinal flexibility, and encourages fluidity in movement.

Day 6-7: Lower Body Preparation

Gradual Leg Stretches (Seated Forward Bend):

Extend your legs for a Seated Forward Bend.

• Inhale, lengthen your spine, and reach towards your toes as you exhale.

• Hold the stretch for 15 seconds, feeling the elongation in your hamstrings.

This exercise stretches the hamstrings, releases tension in the lower back, and promotes leg flexibility.

Core-Strengthening Poses (Seated Boat Pose):

Engage your core with Seated Boat Pose.

• Sit towards the edge of your chair, lift your legs, and keep your back straight.

• Hold the position for 15 seconds, gradually increasing the duration.

This exercise strengthens core muscles, improves balance, and tones abdominal muscles.

Mindfulness Meditation for Relaxation:

Close your eyes, sit comfortably, and focus on your breath. Inhale for four counts, allowing your lungs to fill with air, and exhale for six counts, releasing any tension. Allow thoughts to come and go without attachment. This mindfulness meditation reduces stress, enhances mental clarity, and creates a sense of relaxation and inner calm.

As we build the foundation in Week 1, remember that these practices improve physical and mental health by reducing stress and ensuring a deeper connection between body and mind.

Summary of Week 1:

Day

Focus

Activities

1-2

Establishing the Basics

- Gentle neck and shoulder stretches- Mindful breathing exercises- Introduction to foundational poses

3-5

Upper Body Warm-Up

- Focus on arms, wrists, and hands- Slow introduction to seated twists- Incorporating fluid movements

6-7

Lower Body Preparation

- Gradual leg stretches- Core-strengthening poses- Mindfulness meditation for relaxation

. . .

Week 2: Building Strength and Stability

Day 8-10: Strengthening the Core

Seated Ab Exercises (knee lift):

- Begin seated towards the front of your chair.
- Lift one knee towards your chest, engaging your abdominal muscles.
- Hold for 10 seconds, then switch to the other leg.
- Repeat for ten cycles.

This exercise targets your abdominal muscles, enhancing core strength.

Benefits: Strengthens the core, improves posture, and supports spinal alignment.

Incorporating Twists for Core Stability:

Seated Twist becomes dynamic. Inhale, lengthen your spine, and as you exhale, twist your torso to one side, bringing your opposite hand to the outside of the thigh. Inhale back to the center, then repeat on the other side. Perform ten twists on each side. This exercise enhances core stability and promotes flexibility in the spine.

Benefits: Improves digestion, strengthens obliques, and enhances overall core stability.

Gentle Backbends/Extensions for Spine Health:

In Seated Backbend, gently place your hands on the back of your chair, arching your back. Hold for 15 seconds, feeling the stretch in your chest and spine. This exercise promotes spine health and flexibility and counteracts the effects of prolonged sitting.

Benefits: Increases spine flexibility, relieves tension in the back, and promotes a healthy posture.

Day 11-13: Arm and Leg Strength

Seated Leg Lifts and extensions:

- Sit comfortably in your chair, keeping your back straight.
- Lift one leg at a time, extending it straight in front of you.

- Hold for 10 seconds, then lower it down.
- Repeat with the other leg.
- Perform ten leg lifts on each side.

This exercise targets the quadriceps and improves leg strength.

Benefits: Strengthens leg muscles, enhances flexibility, and improves lower body strength.

Arm Exercises with Added Resistance:

- Grab a resistance band, or use your hands for added resistance.
- Extend your arms in front of you, then pull the band away from your body or press your hands together.
- Repeat for 15 reps.

This exercise targets the biceps, triceps, and shoulders, promoting upper body strength.

Benefits: Toning and strengthening the arms, enhancing shoulder stability, and improving upper body strength.

Chair Squats for Lower Body Strength:

- Stand in front of your chair, feet shoulder-width apart.
- Lower your body into a seated position, as if you were sitting in the chair, then stand back up.
- Perform ten chair squats.

This exercise engages the quadriceps, hamstrings, and glutes, building lower body strength.

Benefits: Strengthens lower body muscles, improves balance, and enhances lower body strength.

Day 14: Integration and Flow

Connecting Movements Seamlessly:

- Integrate the strength you've built into fluid movements.
- Start with a Seated Mountain Pose, transition to a Seated Forward Bend, and then move into a Seated Twist.

• Connect these poses seamlessly, focusing on the smooth transition between each.

• Repeat for five cycles.

This exercise enhances body awareness and uplifts a sense of unity in movement.

Benefits: Improves coordination, enhances flexibility, and promotes a harmonious energy flow throughout the body.

Flowing Through a Short Routine:

• Combine the poses you've learned into a short routine.

• Begin with a Seated Cat-Cow Stretch, move into Seated Leg Lifts, and then transition to Chair Squats.

• Flow through the routine for 3 minutes, synchronizing breath with movement.

This exercise positively affects strength and stability, creating a dynamic and engaging practice.

Benefits: Strengthens multiple muscle groups, improves cardiovascular health, and enhances the overall flow of the practice.

Mindful Meditation on Movement:

• Close your eyes and sit comfortably.

• As you move through the routine, stay present in each pose.

• Focus on the sensations, the breath, and the connection between mind and body.

This meditation on movement develops a sense of mindfulness and presence in your practice.

Benefits: Enhances mental clarity, reduces stress, and deepens the mind-body connection.

As you reach Day 14, celebrate your progress in building strength and stability. Integration and flow are key components of a holistic chair yoga practice. Moving forward, we'll continue to explore new dimensions of your chair yoga practice, enriching your experience. Stay dedicated, and let the flow of movement guide you toward greater strength and harmony.

Summary of Week 2: Building Strength and Stability

Day

Focus
Activities
8-10
Strengthening the Core
- Seated ab exercises- Incorporating twists for core stability- Gentle backbends for spine health
11-13
Arm and Leg Strength
- Seated leg lifts and extensions- Arm exercises with added resistance- Chair squats for lower body strength
14
Integration and Flow
- Connecting movements seamlessly- Flowing through a short routine- Mindful meditation on movement

Week 3: Enhancing Flexibility

Day 15-17: Deepening Stretches

Emphasis on Deeper Stretches for Flexibility:

- Begin with a hamstring stretch, aiming to reach further each time.
- Hold the stretch for 20 seconds, feeling the gradual release.
- Transition to Seated Inner Thigh Stretch
- Hold for 15 seconds on each side.
- Emphasize smooth and controlled movements to deepen your stretches gradually.

Benefits: Increases flexibility in the hamstrings and inner thighs and enhances overall flexibility and range of motion.

Modified Poses for Gradual Progression:

- Modify familiar poses to intensify your stretch.
- In Seated Cat-Cow Stretch, focus on a more pronounced arch and rounding of the spine.
- Hold each position for 15 seconds, then transition smoothly.

This modification allows for a gentle progression in your flexibility journey.

Benefits: Promotes incremental flexibility gains, reduces the risk of strain, and enhances overall mobility.

Introduction to Dynamic Stretching:

- Incorporate dynamic movements into your routine.
- With Seated Leg Swings, swing one leg forward and backward, then switch sides.
- Perform ten swings on each leg.

Dynamic stretching helps warm muscles and improves flexibility by moving joints through a full range of motion.

Benefits: Increases blood flow to muscles, improves flexibility, and prepares the body for deeper stretches.

As you dive into Days 15-17, focus on deepening your stretches and gradually enhancing your flexibility. The modified poses and dynamic stretching will create a more fluid and flexible body. Keep the momentum going, and let the next days bring new dimensions to your chair yoga practice.

Day 18-20: Full Body Flexibility

Integrating Upper and Lower Body Flexibility:

Combine upper and lower body flexibility in a Seated Forward Bend with a Twist. Inhale, lengthen your spine, and as you exhale, reach towards one foot while twisting your torso. Hold for 15 seconds, then switch sides. This integrated approach enhances flexibility in both the upper and lower body.

Benefits: Improves overall body flexibility, enhances spinal mobility, and ensures coordination between upper and lower body movements.

Seated Forward Bends and Twists:

- Dedicate time to Seated Forward Bends and Twists.
- Begin with Advanced Seated Forward Bend, holding for 20 seconds to deepen the stretch in your hamstrings.
- Transition into Seated Twist, holding for 15 seconds on each side.

These poses target multiple muscle groups, improving flexibility throughout the body.

Benefits: Stretches hamstrings and spine, increases flexibility in the back, and promotes overall body suppleness.

Mindful Breathing for Enhanced Flexibility:

- Incorporate mindful breathing into your flexibility routine.
- During each stretch, focus on deep inhalations and exhalations.
- As you breathe out, visualize tension leaving your body.

This mindful breathing practice promotes relaxation and allows for deeper flexibility.

Benefits: Facilitates relaxation, reduces muscle tension, and improves the effectiveness of flexibility exercises.

As you progress through Days 18-20, embrace the synergy of full-body flexibility. Integrating upper and lower body movements and mindful breathing will improve your flexibility. Keep exploring the depths of your practice, and let each stretch bring you closer to a more flexible and resilient you.

Day 21: Flowing Sequence

Combining Flexibility and Fluidity:

- Merge flexibility with fluidity in a flowing sequence.
- Begin with a Seated Mountain Pose, smoothly transition into a Seated Forward Bend, then into a Seated Twist, and finally into Seated Leg Lifts.
- Repeat this sequence for 5 minutes, emphasizing a seamless flow between each pose.

This flowing sequence increases flexibility while promoting a sense of grace and harmony.

Benefits: Results in better overall flexibility, improves coordination, and builds a mindful connection between breath and movement.

Full-Body Stretching Routine:

- Devote this day to a comprehensive full-body stretching routine.
- Utilize Seated Forward Bends, Twists, and dynamic movements like Seated Leg Swings.

• Focus on reaching your full range of motion, holding each stretch for 20 seconds.

This routine provides a holistic stretch, incorporating flexibility across the entire body.

Benefits: Improves overall body flexibility, releases tension in major muscle groups, and enhances joint mobility.

Meditation on Flexibility and Acceptance:

Close your eyes, sit comfortably, and reflect on the flexibility gained throughout this journey. Meditate on the acceptance of where you are in your practice. Inhale acceptance, exhale any judgment. This meditation establishes a positive mindset, improving mental health.

Benefits: Promotes mental clarity, reduces stress, and encourages a positive and accepting attitude towards oneself.

On Day 21, as you immerse yourself in this flowing sequence, let the harmony of flexibility and fluidity guide you. This day goes beyond the physical benefits, focusing on mental health and acceptance. Celebrate your progress, both in body and mind, and carry this newfound sense of flexibility into the upcoming days of your chair yoga practice.

Summary of Week 3: Enhancing Flexibility

Day

Focus

Activities

15-17

Deepening Stretches

- Emphasis on deeper stretches for flexibility- Modified poses for gradual progression- Introduction to dynamic stretching

18-20

Full Body Flexibility

- Integrating upper and lower body flexibility- Seated forward bends and twists- Mindfulness meditation for enhanced flexibility

21

Flowing Sequence

- Combining flexibility and fluidity- Full-body stretching routine- Meditation on flexibility and acceptance

Week 4: Advanced Challenges

Day 22-24: Balancing Poses

Seated Balancing Exercises:

- Challenge your balance with Seated Knee Lifts.
- Sit tall in your chair, lift one knee towards your chest, and hold for 10 seconds.
- Lower it down and switch to the other leg.
- Repeat for ten cycles.

This exercise engages core muscles and challenges stability.

Benefits: Strengthens core muscles, enhances balance, and improves overall stability.

Integrating Mindfulness for Stability:

- Incorporate mindfulness into your balancing practice.
- Focus on your breath and the sensations in your body as you perform the Seated Tree Pose.
- Lift one foot, placing it on the inner thigh or calf of the opposite leg.
- Hold for 15 seconds on each side, maintaining a steady gaze.

This mindfulness-enhanced pose adds an element of stability to your balance practice.

Benefits: Improves concentration, delivers mindfulness, and increases stability in balancing poses.

Day 25-27: Flowing Movements

Full-Body Flowing Sequences:

- Engage in dynamic, full-body-flowing sequences that challenge your coordination and strength.
- Start with Seated Sun Salutations, smoothly transitioning between Seated Mountain Pose, Seated Forward Bend, and Seated Twist.
- Repeat for ten cycles, maintaining a fluid motion.

This flowing sequence addresses flexibility, strength, and overall body awareness.

Benefits: Improves coordination, strengthens major muscle groups, and results in a harmonious flow of movement.

Breathwork for Concentration:

- Incorporate breathwork into your flowing movements.
- Practice Ujjayi breath—inhaling and exhaling through the nose while slightly constricting the back of your throat.
- Sync your breath with each movement in the sequence.

This breathwork enhances concentration, bringing a meditative quality to your practice.

Benefits: Improves focus, reduces stress, and builds the mind-body connection.

The flowing movements not only challenge your physical abilities but also offer an opportunity for mindful concentration. Integrating breathwork creates a clearer sense of presence, allowing your chair yoga practice to evolve into a moving meditation. Keep exploring the fluidity within your movements and breath, and let each sequence bring you closer to a more centered and connected practice.

Day 28: Celebration and Reflection

Celebratory Routine with Favorite Poses:

Today is a celebration of your achievements in chair yoga. Try revisiting your favorite poses from the past 27 days. Whether it's the grounding Seated Mountain Pose, the dynamic Seated Cat-Cow Stretch, or any other pose that resonates with you, take a few moments to enjoy and savor each movement. Repeat your chosen poses for 10 minutes, admiring your progress.

Setting Intentions for Continued Practice

As you conclude this 28-day plan, take a deliberate pause to reflect on the visible impact of your commitment. Setting intentions becomes a powerful tool for shaping the path ahead in the spirit of continued growth.

Reflect on Your Achievements: Take stock of the achievements and breakthroughs you've experienced during these four weeks. Whether it's improved flexibility, enhanced balance, or a newfound sense of calm, acknowledge and celebrate these victories. These milestones are a testament to your dedication and progress.

Identify Areas for Growth: Consider aspects of your chair yoga practice that you'd like to explore further. Is there a specific pose you want to master, a certain area of flexibility you wish to enhance, or perhaps a breathing technique you want to try? Identifying these areas sets the stage for targeted growth in your ongoing journey.

Clarify Your Motivation: What motivates you to continue your chair yoga practice? Clearly articulate your motivations, whether they're the physical benefits, mental clarity, or the overall sense of well-being. Knowing why you show up on your chair for daily yoga practice provides a strong foundation for sustained commitment.

Define Realistic Goals: Set realistic and attainable goals for the upcoming weeks.

These could be daily practices, weekly challenges, or specific milestones you aim to reach. You create a roadmap that inspires and motivates you by breaking down your journey into manageable steps.

Create a Consistent Routine: Establish a consistent practice routine that aligns with your lifestyle. Whether dedicating a specific time each day or incorporating chair yoga into your daily routine, consistency is key to establishing lasting habits.

Visualize Your Future Practice: Envision your chair yoga practice in the future. Picture yourself exploring new poses effortlessly, feeling a sense of strength and balance, and experiencing a deep connection between mind and body. Visualization adds a powerful dimension to your intentions, guiding you toward the practice you aspire to achieve.

Express Gratitude: Take a moment to express gratitude for your time and effort in your fitness. Gratitude acknowledges your journey and sets a positive tone for the days ahead.

Summary of Week 4: Advanced Challenges

Day

Focus

Activities

22-24

Balancing Poses

- Seated balancing exercises- Integrating mindfulness for stability

25-27

Flowing Movements

- Full-body flowing sequences- Breathwork for concentration

28

Celebration and Reflection

- Celebratory routine with favorite poses- Setting intentions for continued practice

Final Words:

In the words of Gene Tunney, "To enjoy the glow of good health, you must exercise." Your 28-day chair yoga journey has been a testament to this wisdom, guiding you through foundational exercises, strength-building challenges, flexibility enhancements, and advanced poses. As you conclude this chapter, achieving better health is not just a distant goal; it is a reality you've actively explored.

Key Takeaways

Progress in Every Pose: Each day brought a new opportunity to progress, whether in foundational poses or advanced challenges. Celebrate the small victories that form the building blocks of a healthier you.

Mind-Body Connection: Chair yoga is not just about physical movement; it's a journey that deepens the connection between your mind and body. The mindful breath, intentional poses, and flowing sequences created a holistic and transformative experience.

As we move to the next chapter, "Step#8: Beyond the Chair", we'll explore how the principles learned within the confines of your chair can be expanded into broader aspects of your life. Chapter 8 opens the door to a broader, more integrated fitness regimen, from mindfulness practices to incorporating yoga into daily activities. So, as you carry the positive results of improved health with you, be ready to extend the benefits beyond the chair, unlocking new dimensions of vitality and balance. Let's surpass the boundaries of your chair yoga practice.

Step #8: Beyond the Chair

"Exercise is amazing, from the inside out. I feel so alive and have more energy." —Vanessa Hudgens.

Vanessa Hudgens perfectly captures the transformative power of exercise. In this chapter, we'll explore the extensive possibilities of chair yoga—beyond the confines of a living room or home routine. Chair yoga need not be a solitary activity; its benefits can extend far beyond physical aspects. Let's break free from the limitations of a stationary chair and discover how chair yoga can become a dynamic and enriching part of your life.

Integrating Chair Yoga into Daily Activities

In the busy routines of our daily lives, finding time for a dedicated yoga session can be a challenge. However, chair yoga offers a unique solution—it can seamlessly integrate into your routine. Here is how you can make chair yoga a companion to your daily activities, improving your fitness, health, and schedule.

Morning Chair Yoga Boost

Begin your day with a burst of energy by incorporating chair yoga into your morning routine. Simple stretches and mindful breathing while seated can set a positive tone for the day. Try the following poses:

Morning Mountain Stretch:

- Sit tall in your chair with your feet flat on the floor.

- Inhale, reaching your arms overhead, stretching towards the ceiling.
- Exhale and lower your arms. Repeat for five breaths.

Seated Forward Fold:

- Sit at the edge of your chair with feet hip-width apart.
- Hinge at your hips, reaching towards your toes.
- Hold for 15-30 seconds, breathing deeply.

Desk Chair Revitalization

For those spending long hours at a desk, chair yoga can be a lifesaver. Discover specific chair yoga poses designed to alleviate tension and strain caused by prolonged sitting. Try these desk-friendly exercises:

Neck Release:

- Sit comfortably and drop your right ear towards your right shoulder.
- Gently hold your head to deepen the stretch.
- Repeat on the other side. Hold each side for 15 seconds.

Seated Twist:

- Sit tall, place your right hand on the outside of your left knee.
- Twist gently to the left, looking over your shoulder.
- Hold for 15-30 seconds, then switch sides.

Chair Yoga Breaks

Even amid a hectic schedule, taking short breaks for chair yoga can enhance your focus and productivity. Learn a set of quick, effective exercises that can be done during your coffee break or between tasks:

Seated Cat-Cow Stretch:

- Sit tall, and place your hands on your knees.
- Inhale, arch your back (cow), exhale, and round your spine (cat).

- Repeat for 1-2 minutes.

Chair Pigeon Pose:

- Sit at the edge of your chair and cross your right ankle over your left knee.
- Sit tall, feeling a stretch in your right hip.
- Hold for 15-30 seconds, then switch sides.

Evening Relaxation Routine

As the day winds down, wind down with chair yoga. Here are a few relaxing poses and breathing exercises that can help release the tension accumulated throughout the day:

Seated Butterfly Stretch:

- Sit comfortably with the soles of your feet together.
- Hold your feet and gently flap your knees.
- Breathe deeply, holding for 1-2 minutes.

Deep Breathing Exercise:

- Sit tall, close your eyes.
- Inhale deeply for a count of 4, hold for 4, and exhale for 4.
- Repeat for 5 minutes.

Daily Activity Fusion

Finally, explore the concept of fusing chair yoga with other daily activities. Whether waiting for your commute, standing in line, or watching TV, there are ample opportunities to incorporate chair yoga seamlessly into your day. Consider these practical tips:

Waiting Warrior:

- Stand with feet hip-width apart.
- Lift arms overhead, clasping hands.
- Take a deep breath, stretching up. Hold for 15 seconds.

TV Time Toe Taps:

- Sit on the edge of your chair.
- Lift your legs and tap your toes in front of you.
- Increase speed for a mini cardio boost during your favorite show.

Remember, the key is to make chair yoga a natural part of your day, adapting it to fit your lifestyle and schedule.

Chair Yoga for Travel and Commuting

Traveling and commuting can often be stressful, but with chair yoga, you can transform these moments into opportunities for relaxation and self-care. Whether on a long flight, a train, or simply commuting to work, make the most of your time and rejuvenate your body and mind with these chair yoga techniques.

In-Flight Serenity

Airplanes can be cramped, and long flights can leave you feeling stiff and tired. Try these chair yoga poses to enhance your in-flight experience:

Ankle Circles: Enhance Circulation

- Lift your feet off the floor, drawing circles with your toes.
- Rotate your ankles clockwise for ten rotations, then counterclockwise.
- This simple exercise promotes blood circulation, preventing stiffness.

Seated Spinal Twist: Alleviate Tension

- Sit tall and cross your right hand to your left knee.
- Twist gently to the left, looking over your shoulder.
- Hold for 15-30 seconds, then switch sides.
- Relieve tension in your spine and keep your back feeling limber.

Commuting Calm

Whether you're driving, taking the bus, or commuting on a train, chair yoga can help you make the most of your travel time:

Steering Wheel Shoulder Stretch: Ease Upper Body Tension

- While stopped, place your right hand on the top of the steering wheel.
- Gently turn your body to the right, feeling a stretch in your shoulders.
- Hold for 15 seconds, then switch sides.
- Alleviate tension in your neck and shoulders after a day's work.

Seated Chest Opener: Improve Posture

- Sit tall and interlace your fingers behind your back.
- Open your chest, squeezing your shoulder blades together.
- Hold for 15-30 seconds, maintaining steady breaths.
- Counteract the effects of hunching over screens during your commute.

Hotel Room Relaxation

Traveling often involves spending nights away from home. Turn your hotel room into a sanctuary for relaxation with these chair yoga poses:

Bedside Forward Fold: Release Tension Before Bed

- Sit on the edge of the bed with your feet flat on the floor.
- Hinge at your hips, reaching towards the floor.
- Hold for 15-30 seconds, breathing deeply.
- Promote relaxation and prepare your body for a restful night.

Chair-Supported Tree Pose: Find Balance

- Stand beside a chair, holding the back for support.
- Lift your right foot and place it on your inner left thigh.
- Hold for balance and stability. Switch sides after 30 seconds.
- Improve balance and flexibility in the comfort of your hotel room.

Communal Commuting

If commuting is a shared experience, consider building a chair yoga community. Share simple exercises with fellow travelers or coworkers to create a positive, supportive environment:

Shared Shoulder Stretch

- Sit back-to-back with a partner.
- Interlace your fingers and stretch your arms, feeling a gentle shoulder stretch.
- Communicate and adjust for comfort.
- Create a sense of connection and camaraderie during the commute.

Communal Mindful Breathing

- Inhale for a count of 4, exhale for 4.
- Encourage others to join in, creating a calming atmosphere during the commute.
- Practice mindfulness and reduce stress for everyone on the journey.

Embrace the mobility that chair yoga provides, making your journeys more enjoyable and your destinations more satisfying. Whether on a plane, train, or automobile, chair yoga can transform travel time into an opportunity for rejuvenation.

Sharing Chair Yoga with Friends and Family

Chair yoga doesn't have to be a solo experience; it can be a delightful and social activity when shared with friends and family. This section will highlight how you can introduce chair yoga to your loved ones, making it a bonding activity that promotes health for everyone involved.

Family-Friendly Chair Yoga Sessions

Gather the family for an enjoyable chair yoga session that caters to all age groups. Here are some family-friendly chair yoga poses to get you started:

Chair Cat-Cow Stretch

- Sit on the edge of the chair, hands on your knees.
- Inhale, arch your back (cow), exhale, round your spine (cat).

- Repeat for a few minutes, encouraging family members to join in.
- Share a laugh as you explore the motions together, making it a light and enjoyable experience.

Partner Seated Twist

- Sit back-to-back with a family member.
- Twist to one side while your partner twists to the opposite side.
- Hold for 15 seconds, then switch sides.
- Strengthen the connection with your partner as you support each other in this shared stretching pose.

Chair Yoga Social Gatherings

Host chair yoga sessions with friends to combine fitness and socializing. Make it an event with these engaging chair yoga activities:

Chair Yoga Picnic

- Find a comfortable outdoor space and bring chairs.
- Lead friends through a series of seated stretches and poses.
- Follow up with healthy snacks for a wholesome experience.
- Establish a sense of community by connecting in a natural climate.

Chair Yoga and Chat

- Create a virtual chair yoga session with friends.
- Use video calls to guide each other through chair yoga exercises.
- Discuss your experiences and catch up while staying active.
- Enhance the virtual connection, making it a regular and cherished social activity.

Chair Yoga Parties

Make chair yoga a feature at parties and special occasions for a unique and health-conscious celebration:

Birthday Chair Yoga

- Arrange chairs in a circle and guide guests through celebratory poses.
- Incorporate fun elements like musical chairs with a yoga twist.
- End with a relaxation pose for a serene birthday celebration.
- Create lasting memories by combining the joy of celebration with the benefits of chair yoga.

Office Chair Yoga Breaks

- Introduce chair yoga breaks during work events or conferences.
- Conduct short chair yoga sessions to refresh and energize participants.
- Enhance team bonding while promoting health.
- Ensure a positive workplace culture by integrating chair yoga into professional gatherings.

Chair Yoga Challenges

Transform chair yoga into a friendly competition with challenges that promote fitness and camaraderie:

Chair Yoga Pose Challenge

- Create a list of chair yoga poses.
- Challenge friends or family to replicate the poses.
- Share pictures or videos, establishing a sense of achievement.
- Encourage creativity and laughter as participants take on the challenge together.

Monthly Chair Yoga Marathon

- Set a monthly goal for the number of chair yoga sessions.
- Encourage friends and family to join in and track their progress.
- Celebrate milestones and achievements together.
- Establish a sense of ongoing commitment to health, creating a supportive community.

Sharing chair yoga with friends and family promotes physical health and strengthens the bonds between individuals. Whether it's a family session, a social gathering, a party feature, or a friendly challenge, chair yoga can become a shared experience that brings joy and health to all involved.

Chair Yoga in Group Settings

Chair yoga isn't just an individual practice; it's a fantastic way to bring people together in a group setting. This section discusses the benefits of chair yoga in a social environment, exploring how it enhances physical health and promotes shared experiences.

The Power of Social Exercise

Chair yoga in group settings goes beyond the individual benefits; it becomes a shared activity that strengthens social bonds. Engaging in exercise together creates a supportive atmosphere, encouraging participants to connect physically and emotionally. The shared experience of stretching and breathing in unison creates a sense of unity and shared purpose, breaking down social barriers and creating a positive environment.

In group settings, participants can feed off each other's energy, making the chair yoga session more dynamic and enjoyable. The collective motivation elevates the experience, making individuals more likely to adhere to a regular practice. Social exercise, like chair yoga in a group, can be a powerful tool for building a community centered around better health.

Chair Yoga Social Gatherings for Seniors

Imagine turning your gatherings with other seniors into uplifting chair yoga sessions, creating moments of joy and positivity. Whether it's a seniors' club meeting, a delightful retirement community event, or a heartwarming family reunion, infusing chair yoga into these moments adds a special touch to the experience.

Seniors' Club Chair Yoga Gathering:

- Create a cozy setup with chairs, ensuring everyone has a comfortable spot.
- Begin with gentle warm-ups, like seated neck stretches and shoulder rolls.
- Guide club members through age-appropriate chair yoga poses, emphasizing relaxation.
- Encourage sharing stories and laughter during the session, promoting a sense of camaraderie.
- Conclude with a soothing breathing exercise, leaving everyone refreshed and connected.

Retirement Community Chair Yoga Hour:

- Schedule a regular chair yoga session for the retirement community, ensuring it's easily accessible.
- Start with simple seated movements, such as gentle twists, to ease into the practice.
- Incorporate playful activities like chair-based arm lifts to enhance strength and flexibility.
- Create a supportive atmosphere where everyone feels included and valued.
- End the session with a relaxation pose, allowing seniors to unwind and socialize.

Family Reunion Chair Yoga for Seniors:

- Arrange chairs in a circle, creating a communal space for family members.
- Share memories as you guide seniors through gentle poses like seated side stretches.
- Embrace laughter and storytelling during the session, making it a memorable family experience.
- Conclude with a short meditation, promoting peace and mental clarity.
- Establish chair yoga as a tradition within the family. It will spread a healthy lifestyle across generations.

Chair Yoga in the Workplace

Transforming the workplace through chair yoga can significantly impact employee morale and overall health. These sessions offer employees a chance to unwind, take a mental break, and rejuvenate during the hustle of the workday.

Midday Mindful Moments:

- Schedule brief chair yoga sessions for employees during midday breaks.
- Focus on gentle stretches and calming breath exercises to ease tension.
- Enhance concentration and reduce workplace stress, ensuring a more focused and productive work environment.

- Prioritize the health of employees by establishing a positive workplace atmosphere.

Chair Yoga for Team Bonding:

- Incorporate chair yoga into team-building activities to create a unique bonding experience.
- Facilitate collaborative chair yoga exercises that encourage communication and teamwork.
- Strengthen team dynamics by creating a sense of unity and shared healthy activities.
- Improve workplace relationships, creating a supportive and healthy work culture.

Office Energizer Breaks:

- Use short chair yoga breaks as energizers during the workday.
- Include invigorating chair-based movements to refresh employees.
- Boost overall morale by creating a workplace environment that values productivity and fitness.
- Promote a culture of health and collaboration, making chair yoga an integral part of the work routine.

Chair Yoga for Stress Relief:

- Offer specific chair yoga sessions focused on stress relief.
- Incorporate calming poses and mindfulness techniques to alleviate workplace pressures.
- Provide employees with practical tools to manage stress. It will help promote their mental health.
- Nurture a positive work environment by addressing and alleviating stressors.

By infusing chair yoga into the workplace routine, employees benefit physically and experience improved mental health. It's about creating a workplace that values health, collaboration, and the overall happiness of its employees.

Chair Yoga Classes and Workshops

Consider organizing or attending chair yoga classes and workshops in your local community. This creates a structured environment where individuals can come together to learn and practice chair yoga under the guidance of an instructor.

Community Chair Yoga Class:

- Partner with local community centers or wellness studios to offer chair yoga classes.
- Create a space for community members to gather, learn, and exercise together.
- Promote a sense of shared health within the community.

Chair Yoga Workshop for Beginners:

- Host workshops to introduce chair yoga to beginners.
- Provide detailed instructions on poses and breathing techniques.
- Create a supportive learning environment, encouraging participants to share their experiences.

Practicing chair yoga in group settings enriches the exercise experience by adding a social dimension. Whether in community events, family reunions, workplace wellness programs, or organized classes, the shared practice of chair yoga strengthens bonds, promotes a sense of community, and improves the overall health of individuals.

Connecting with Fellow Chair Yoga Practitioners

Chair yoga becomes even more enriching when practiced alongside like-minded individuals. This section explores avenues to connect with fellow chair yoga practitioners online and in real life. Discover the benefits of community support, shared experiences, and the joy of practicing chair yoga together.

Online Chair Yoga Communities

The digital era has opened up endless possibilities for connecting with fellow chair yoga enthusiasts. Joining online communities provides a platform to share experiences, seek advice, and celebrate milestones:

Social Media Groups:

- Explore chair yoga groups on platforms like Facebook and Instagram.
- Share your progress, ask questions, and engage in discussions.

- Connect with practitioners worldwide, expanding your chair yoga community.

Virtual Chair Yoga Classes:

- Attend live virtual chair yoga classes or webinars.
- Interact with instructors and fellow participants in real-time.
- Make connections by regularly participating and engaging in online discussions.

Local Meetup Groups

Connecting with local chair yoga practitioners in real life can be a rewarding experience. Look for or create meetup groups that gather for regular chair yoga sessions or related activities:

Public Park Gatherings:

- Organize chair yoga meetups in local parks or community spaces.
- Invite individuals to join for a shared outdoor practice.
- Strengthen community bonds and enjoy the benefits of practicing in nature.

Community Center Classes:

- Check with local community centers for chair yoga classes.
- Attend classes to meet practitioners and build connections.
- Create a sense of community while improving health and fitness.

Chair Yoga Events and Retreats

Participating in chair yoga events and retreats provides an immersive experience, developing deep connections with other practitioners:

Chair Yoga Workshops:

- Attend workshops conducted by experienced chair yoga instructors.
- Learn new techniques, share insights, and connect with others.

• Enjoy a supportive environment focused on mutual growth and wellness.

Wellness Retreats:

• Explore chair yoga-focused wellness retreats.

• Immerse yourself in an environment dedicated to health and relaxation.

• Connect with practitioners on a deeper level while enjoying a holistic wellness experience.

Chair Yoga Challenges and Competitions

Engage in chair yoga challenges and competitions to connect with practitioners who share a competitive spirit. These events can be both online and in-person:

Online Challenges:

• Participate in online chair yoga challenges on social media.

• Connect with others by sharing your progress and experiences.

• Arrange friendly competition while building a supportive virtual community.

Local Competitions:

• Join or organize chair yoga competitions in your local community.

• Connect with practitioners who enjoy a more competitive aspect of yoga.

• Celebrate achievements together and create a sense of shared accomplishment.

Connecting with fellow chair yoga practitioners, whether online or in real life, enhances the overall experience. By being part of a supportive community, individuals can share their journey, gain inspiration, and find joy in practicing chair yoga together.

Final Words

As we conclude this exploration of chair yoga beyond the chair, let's circle back to Vanessa Hudgens' insightful words, "Exercise is amazing, from the inside out. I feel so alive and have more energy." Chair yoga indeed encapsulates this sentiment, and in this chapter, we've delved into taking this practice to new heights—beyond the confines of a stationary chair. The possibilities are expansive, from integrating chair yoga into your daily routine to sharing the experience with friends, family, coworkers and even fellow practitioners worldwide.

Key Takeaways

Chair Yoga is Inclusive and Adaptable: The beauty of chair yoga lies in its adaptability. It seamlessly integrates into various aspects of your life, becoming a flexible and accessible wellness tool for individuals of all ages and abilities.

Community Amplifies the Experience: Whether connecting virtually or in real life, the communal aspect of chair yoga enhances the overall experience. Sharing the chair yoga practice creates a supportive environment that promotes motivation, connection, and the joy of shared improvements.

As you venture beyond the chair and embrace chair yoga in its multiple forms, may this chapter inspire you to not only enhance your health but also to incorporate chair yoga into your daily life. Embrace the positive change, and let chair yoga be a constant companion in pursuing holistic health and vitality.

* * *

TAKE A MOMENT TO PLEASE LEAVE A REVIEW

Yoga lovers, ever considered how your review of "The Ultimate Illustrated Guide to Chair Yoga for Seniors Over 60" could inspire someone to embrace a more active, joyful life? Your words might just be the push they need to start their own journey into chair yoga, showing that staying active knows no age.

Share your story. Whether the book boosted your mobility or made you giggle during a tricky pose, your honest feedback can light the way for others.

Simply head to amzn.to/4aTg2n5 or scan the QR code to leave your review.

USA

UK

CAN

Your insights can spark change, motivating others towards a healthier life and connecting you with a community that cherishes wellness.

Let's spread the joy of chair yoga together. Your review isn't just feedback; it's an act of kindness and support. Share your experience, one review at a time.

Conclusion

Chair Yoga for a Vibrant Life

"The Ultimate Illustrated Guide to Chair Yoga for Seniors Over 60" highlighted the transformative power of chair yoga—a practice that transcends age, abilities, and limitations. At its core, chair yoga is more than just a series of movements; it's a holistic approach to better health and fitness, creating a deep connection between the mind and body.

Key Takeaways:

1) Inclusivity and Adaptability:

We discovered that chair yoga is a practice for all. It transcends age and fitness levels, inviting everyone to journey toward improved health. The inclusivity takeaway is not just a concept; it's a living reality of chair yoga, demonstrated through accessible poses and a mindset that values each individual's unique abilities.

2) Mind-Body Connection:

The mind-body connection became our guiding light as we explored the Fundamental Poses. Chair yoga is not merely about physical exercise; it's a mindful exploration where each pose promotes a deeper connection between your mind and body. The integration of mindfulness in every movement, highlighted in every chapter, has become a cornerstone of this holistic practice.

3) Community Amplification:

Chair yoga is not a solitary endeavor but a communal experience. In Beyond the Chair, we discovered how the practice extends beyond the personal level to community amplification. Sharing chair yoga experiences virtually or in real life makes it even more joyful. This aspect reinforces the importance of building a supportive community that motivates and multiplies the happiness of shared wellness practices.

4) Accessible Wellness:

The Beginner Poses Mastery brought us face-to-face with the foundational elements of chair yoga. The accessible wellness became evident as we explored 25 beginner poses designed for individuals of all abilities. Chair yoga is not just a physical exercise; it's an accessible avenue for everyone to start their fitness journey.

5) Consistency is Key:

In Mastering Beginner Poses, we introduced a daily routine blueprint, emphasizing the importance of consistency. The provided daily planner empowers you to seamlessly integrate chair yoga into your life, offering a structured routine that accommodates warm-up, main poses, and cool-down exercises in 10 minutes. The importance of regular engagement with poses, coupled with mindful reflection, became evident in this takeaway.

6) Balancing Act:

Mastering Intermediate Poses revealed the delicate balance that defines intermediate chair yoga. From Seated Warrior III to Quad Stretches, we learned that the balancing act is not just about refining simplicity but embracing the challenges of complexity. Each pose contributes to a harmonious blend of strength and flexibility, representing the essence of mastering intermediate poses.

7) Progress is a Journey:

In Mastering Advanced Poses, we discovered that progress is a slow process. It's not about achieving perfection overnight but a gradual exploration of each pose, appreciating the progress along the way. The mindful exploration of advanced poses became the essence of this key takeaway.

8) Mind-Body Connection Deepens:

In The 28-Day Challenge, we emphasized that mind-body connection is not a static concept. It deepens with each day, whether in foundational poses or advanced challenges. Celebrating the small victories formed the building blocks of a healthier you.

9) Chair Yoga Beyond the Chair:

In the final chapter, Beyond the Chair, we explored the expansive possibilities that chair yoga offers. The adaptability of chair yoga seamlessly integrates into various aspects of life, becoming a flexible wellness tool. The success extends beyond the chair; we explored how to incorporate chair yoga into daily routines, social connections, and a broader, more integrated fitness journey.

Real-Life Success Stories:

Let's draw inspiration from real-life success stories of people benefiting from Chair yoga. Carol Tager, at the age of 86, experienced life-changing benefits through chair yoga at the Roseville Health & Wellness Center. Chair yoga improved her posture, reduced joint pain from arthritis, increased flexibility, lowered stress, deepened her sleep, and improved core strength. Her story is a testament to the transformative power of chair yoga in enhancing overall well-being, irrespective of age. And it's not unique; it's one of hundreds and thousands of testimonials showcasing the power of chair yoga. (*Success Stories | Roseville Health & Wellness*, n.d.)

Seize the Moment:

With this book's knowledge and practicality, you stand on the threshold of a healthier, more fulfilling life. As we conclude, this is not just about exercise; it's about enjoying the glow of good health from the inside out. Each small victory, every mindful breath, creates a healthier you. Let chair yoga be your guide to unlocking new dimensions of vitality and balance.

Don't let this newfound knowledge go to waste. It's time to proceed in your chair yoga practice, no matter your reason, skill level, or personal needs. The power to enhance your physical health is now within your grasp.

Consider incorporating chair yoga into your daily routine. Use the dedicated space you've created, explore fundamental poses, and consistently progress through the stages. Let chair yoga become an integral part of your life, enhancing not only your physical health but also your mental and emotional well-being.

Share Your Feedback:

If this book has resonated with you and positively impacted your life, we'd love to hear about it. Share your experiences, and consider leaving a review. Your feedback will motivate others to start their chair yoga practice and help us create resources catering to seniors' unique needs.

In closing, may chair yoga be your constant companion in pursuing holistic health and vitality.

Resources

American Heart Association. (2014, September 1). Warm up, cool down. Retrieved from https://www.heart.org/en/healthy-living/fitness/fitness-basics/warm-up-cool-down

Aston Gardens. (n.d.). Great benefits of chair yoga for seniors. Retrieved from https://www.astongardens.com/senior-living-blog/great-benefits-of-chair-yoga-for-seniors/

Autonomous. (n.d.). 15 seated stretching exercises. Retrieved from https://www.autonomous.ai/ourblog/15-seated-stretching-exercises

Better Health Channel. (n.d.). Exercise safety. Retrieved from https://www.betterhealth.vic.gov.au/health/healthyliving/exercise-safety

BetterMe. (n.d.). Advanced chair yoga poses. Retrieved from https://betterme.world/articles/advanced-chair-yoga-poses/

Bharshankar, J. R., Bharshankar, R. N., Deshpande, V. N., Kaore, S. B., & Gosavi, G. B. (2003). Effect of yoga on cardiovascular system in subjects above 40 years. Indian Journal of Physiology and Pharmacology, 47(2), 202–206. Retrieved from https://pubmed.ncbi.nlm.nih.gov/15255625/

Buffalo Spree. (n.d.). Chair yoga. Retrieved from https://www.buffalospree.com/style_living/healthy_lifestyles/chair-yoga/article_4bfde06e-dd1e-11ec-a298-0fb3e1e3bd81.html

Chopra. (n.d.). 4 advanced meditation techniques and tools to deepen your practice. Retrieved from https://chopra.com/blogs/meditation/4-advanced-meditation-techniques-and-tools-to-deepen-your-practice

ElderGym. (n.d.). Chair exercises for seniors. Retrieved from https://eldergym.com/chair-exercises-for-seniors/

Exercises for pain-free hands. (2013, January 24). Harvard Health. Retrieved from https://www.health.harvard.edu/pain/exercises-for-pain-free-hands

Flowithme. (2020, October 30). Chair yoga as a natural relief from arthritis pain | chair yoga | pain | arthritis | yoga. Retrieved from https://www.flowithme.com/post/chair-yoga-for-students-with-arthritis

Gear Baron. (n.d.). Best yoga chairs. Retrieved from https://gearbaron.com/articles/best-yoga-chairs/

GoodRx. (n.d.). Chair yoga. Retrieved from https://www.goodrx.com/well-being/movement-exercise/chair-yoga

Greatist. (n.d.). Chair squats. Retrieved from https://greatist.com/fitness/chair-squats

Harvard Health Publishing. (2013, January 24). Exercises for pain free hands. Retrieved from https://www.health.harvard.edu/pain/exercises-for-pain-free-hands

Healthline. (2022, February 15). How to engage your core: Steps, muscles worked, and more. Retrieved from https://www.healthline.com/nutrition/how-to-engage-your-core

Kripalu. (n.d.). Surprising benefits of chair yoga. Retrieved from https://kripalu.org/resources/surprising-benefits-chair-yoga

Lakes at Litchfield Senior Living. (n.d.). Chair yoga. Retrieved from https://lakeseminoleseniorliving.com/blog/chair-yoga/

Lifeline. (n.d.). Core exercises for seniors. Retrieved from https://www.lifeline.ca/en/resources/core-exercises-for-seniors/

Lifespan. (2020, February 12). Yoga and meditation. Retrieved from https://meditation.studio/yoga-and-meditation/

LinkedIn. (n.d.). Creating a safe & hygienic workout environment. Retrieved from https://www.linkedin.com/pulse/creating-safe-hygienic-workout-environment-clearlypremier

Lockton Personal Training Insurance. (n.d.). How to create a friendly & safe environment. Retrieved from https://locktonpersonaltraininginsurance.com/how-to-create-friendly-safe-environment/

ManFlowYoga. (n.d.). Challenging yoga exercises you can do on a chair. Retrieved from https://manflowyoga.com/blog/challenging-yoga-exercises-you-can-do-on-a-chair/

Mary Dana Yoga. (n.d.). Chair yoga: Where do I start? A prop buying guide. Retrieved from https://www.marydanayoga.com/post/chair-yoga-where-do-i-start-a-prop-buying-guide

Medical News Today. (n.d.). Chair yoga for seniors. Retrieved from https://www.medicalnewstoday.com/articles/chair-yoga-for-seniors

Monday Campaigns. (n.d.). 3 chair yoga poses for all fitness levels Monday. Retrieved from https://www.mondaycampaigns.org/move-it-monday/3-chair-yoga-poses-fitness-levels-monday

National Center for Biotechnology Information. (n.d.). Why seated yoga poses are good for you. Retrieved from https://www.ncbi.nlm.nih.gov/pmc/articles/PMC10094373/

Nourish Yoga Training. (n.d.). How to chair yoga. Retrieved from https://nourishyogatraining.com/how-to-chair-yoga/

OnePeloton. (n.d.). Chair yoga. Retrieved from https://www.onepeloton.com/blog/chair-yoga/

Park, J., McCaffrey, R., Newman, D., Liehr, P., & Ouslander, J. G. (2016). A pilot randomized controlled trial of the effects of chair yoga on pain and physical function among community-dwelling older adults with lower extremity osteoarthritis. Journal of the American Geriatrics Society, 65(3), 592–597. https://doi.org/10.1111/jgs.14717

Performance Health. (n.d.). Chair yoga for seniors: 6 exercises to maintain strength and flexibility. Retrieved from https://www.performancehealth.com/articles/chair-yoga-for-seniors-6-exercises-to-maintain-strength-and-flexibility

Resources

PureGym. (n.d.). Chair yoga exercises for beginners and seniors. Retrieved from https://www.puregym.com/blog/chair-yoga-exercises-for-beginners-and-seniors/

Release Muscle Therapy. (n.d.). Chair sits squats. Retrieved from https://releasemuscletherapy.com/chair-sits-squats/

Rise and Vibe Yoga. (n.d.). Chair yoga. Retrieved from https://www.riseandvibeyoga.com/blog/chair-yoga

Schettler, R. (2021, December 23). 14 modifications for common yoga poses that you've probably never seen before. Yoga Journal. Retrieved from https://www.yogajournal.com/poses/14-modifications-for-common-yoga-poses/

Scripps Health. (n.d.). 7 tips to get you exercising consistently. Retrieved from [insert URL]

Shinners, R. (2016, April 8). 15 quotes that will inspire you to be healthier. Woman's Day. Retrieved from https://www.womansday.com/health-fitness/g2318/healthy-lifestyle-quotes/

SilverSneakers. (n.d.). 4 chair exercises. Retrieved from https://www.silversneakers.com/blog/4-chair-exercises/

SilverSneakers. (n.d.). 7 standing exercises for core strength. Retrieved from https://www.silversneakers.com/blog/7-standing-exercises-for-core-strength/

SilverSneakers. (n.d.). 10 total-body stretches you can do from a chair. Retrieved from https://www.silversneakers.com/blog/10-total-body-stretches-you-can-do-from-a-chair/

SoundCloud. (n.d.). Chair yoga for seniors over 60 quick simple 10-minute chair yoga exercises with step-by-s. Retrieved from https://soundcloud.com/user-884542757/chair-yoga-for-seniors-over-60-quick-simple-10-minute-chair-yoga-exercises-with-step-by-s

SparkPeople. (n.d.). Exercise 126. Retrieved from https://www.sparkpeople.com/resource/exercises.asp?exercise=126

Staff, W. (2019, March 27). Centenarian Toni Stahl credits family and being active for longevity. WNKY News 40 Television. Retrieved from https://www.wnky.com/centenarian-toni-stahl-credits-family-and-being-active-for-longevity/

Stamina Products. (n.d.). 10 ways to track fitness progress. Retrieved from https://staminaproducts.com/blog/10-ways-to-track-fitness-progress/

StartStanding. (n.d.). Best chair yoga poses for back pain. Retrieved from https://www.startstanding.org/sitting-back-pain/best-chair-yoga-poses-for-back-pain/

Step2Health. (n.d.). Seated balance exercises for seniors: 5 moves to try. Retrieved from https://step2health.com/blogs/news/seated-balance-exercises-for-seniors-5-moves-to-try

The Access Healthcare. (n.d.). Chair yoga for seniors. Retrieved from https://theaccesshealthcare.com/blogs/chair-yoga-for-seniors

The Arthritis Foundation. (n.d.). 7 dynamic warm-ups. Retrieved from https://www.arthritis.org/health-wellness/healthy-living/physical-activity/other-activities/7-dynamic-warm-ups

TODAY. (n.d.). Chair yoga poses. Retrieved from https://www.today.com/health/diet-fitness/chair-yoga-poses-rcna101778

Tummee. (n.d.). Chair yoga poses. Retrieved from https://www.tummee.com/yoga-poses/chair-yoga-poses

Tummee. (n.d.). Senior chair yoga back pain. Retrieved from https://www.tummee.com/yoga-sequences/senior-chair-yoga-back-pain

UMN Extension. (n.d.). Healthy and fit on the go: Basic yoga. Retrieved from https://extension.umn.edu/physical-activity/healthy-and-fit-go-basic-yoga

WellDefined. (n.d.). 10-minute all-levels office chair yoga routine from Hilton Head Health. Retrieved from https://welldefined.com/wd-tv/10-minute-all-levels-office-chair-yoga-routine-from-hilton-head-health/

Women's Health Network. (n.d.). Chair yoga poses. Retrieved from https://www.womenshealthnetwork.com/other-womens-health/chair-yoga-poses/

Woman's Day. (2016, April 8). 15 quotes that will inspire you to be healthier. Retrieved from https://www.womansday.com/health-fitness/g2318/healthy-lifestyle-quotes/

Yao, C.-T., & Tseng, C.-H. (2019). Effectiveness of chair yoga for improving the functional fitness and well-being of female community-dwelling older adults with low physical activities. Topics in Geriatric Rehabilitation, 35(4), 248–254. https://doi.org/10.1097/tgr.0000000000000242

Yao, C.-T., Lee, B.-O., Hong, H., & Su, Y.-C. (2023). Effect of chair yoga therapy on functional fitness and daily life activities among older female adults with knee osteoarthritis in Taiwan: A quasi-experimental study. Healthcare, 11(7), 1024. https://doi.org/10.3390/healthcare11071024

Yoga International. (n.d.). A yoga practice for connection. Retrieved from https://yogainternational.com/article/view/a-yoga-practice-for-connection

Yoga Journal. (n.d.). Chair yoga. Retrieved from https://www.yogajournal.com/poses/chair-yoga/

Yoga Journal. (n.d.). Modify chair pose. Retrieved from https://www.yogajournal.com/poses/modify-chair-pose/

Yoga Room Hawaii. (n.d.). 7 amazing yoga breath exercises for breathwork beginners. Retrieved from https://www.yogaroomhawaii.com/blog/7-amazing-yoga-breath-exercises-for-breathwork-beginners

YogaUOnline. (n.d.). Banish the slouch: Chair yoga for healthier posture. Retrieved from https://yogauonline.com/yoga-practice-teaching-tips/yoga-practice-tips/banish-the-slouch-chair-yoga-for-healthier-posture

YouTube. (n.d.). Chair yoga for seniors over 60 quick simple 10-minute chair yoga exercises with step-by-s. Retrieved from https://www.youtube.com/watch?v=OMmcmO3ejTY

YouTube. (n.d.). I7LofxyxwEc. Retrieved from https://www.youtube.com/watch?v=I7LofxyxwEc

YouTube. (n.d.). llFzAvawkjE. Retrieved from https://www.youtube.com/watch?v=llFzAvawkjE

YouTube. (n.d.). 2rwCdGW-7q8. Retrieved from https://www.youtube.com/watch?v=2rwCdGW-7q8

www.ingramcontent.com/pod-product-compliance
Lightning Source LLC
Chambersburg PA
CBHW051731020426
42333CB00014B/1250
9781738268719